The Grammatical Nature of Minimal Structures

The Grammatical Nature of Minimal Structures: Impoverishment of Grammatical Features in a Non-fluent Aphasic Speaker

By

Maria Garraffa

CAMBRIDGE SCHOLARS

PUBLISHING

The Grammatical Nature of Minimal Structures:
Impoverishment of Grammatical Features in a Non-fluent Aphasic Speaker,
by Maria Garraffa

This book first published 2011

Cambridge Scholars Publishing

12 Back Chapman Street, Newcastle upon Tyne, NE6 2XX, UK

British Library Cataloguing in Publication Data
A catalogue record for this book is available from the British Library

ISBN (10): 1-4438-2982-X, ISBN (13): 978-1-4438-2982-3

This small study is dedicated to Maria, whose approach to the investigation of her language impairment has been one of lively curiosity, and to Rosa, Ada and Gian Marco, with whom I share my most intimate thoughts.

TABLE OF CONTENTS

ABSTRACT

The present study is an examination of an Italian aphasic speaker (M.R.) with non-fluent speech following a focal lesion in the left hemisphere.

We develop an explanation of M.R.'s language impairment compatible with theories of generative syntax and with some observations on sentence parsing strategies. The explanatory framework we adopt considers the grammar to be an *integral* part of language processing.

A series of experiments was run across modalities (production, comprehension and grammaticality judgments), with the aim of defining impaired linguistic structures grammatically. Results of the various experiments show selective impairment in some configurations involving object movement in relative clauses, in Wh-questions and in clitic object constructions.

Comprehension deficit for non-canonical sentences has been attested since Caramazza and Zurif's seminal work (1976). In the present case study a similar subject/object asymmetry emerges in interrogative sentence production, which has been found to be impaired for object movement of animate arguments. Interesting data was obtained testing attraction effects with clitics and prepositional modifiers. M.R. does not manifest attraction effects if a clitic object is a potential intervener for the relevant agreement relation; prepositional modifiers induce significant attraction effects.

This case study lends support to the hypothesis that the linguistic deficit presented is an impoverishment of procedural capacities. This impoverishment is grammatically driven, and it manifests itself in reduced syntactic structures. M.R.'s linguistic competence is not different to that of a speaker with a non-impaired grammatical system. M.R. has the capacity to analyze sentences respecting syntactic phrase structures, but not in the way normal speakers do. Crucially, this approach to aphasia does not assume the existence of a specific grammatical deficit, as in so-called agrammatism.

FOREWORD

On the connections between theoretical linguistics and the experimental study of pathologies.

This book puts together two distinct, broad domains of inquiry on language. The first is the detailed formal modeling of linguistic capacities, stemming from theoretical and comparative linguistics; the second is the experimental study of language pathologies, which is in turn a particular chapter of the large endeavor of the experimental investigation of the linguistic abilities in normal and special circumstances, and of how such abilities are expressed in the human brain.

Why should theoretical linguists and specialists of experimental approaches interact in joint research projects of this kind? I think such interdisciplinary collaborations are in the mutual interests of both disciplinary domains.

From the viewpoint of experimental psycholinguistics, neurolinguistics, clinical linguistics (as well as the experimental study of first and second language acquisition), precise formal linguistic models are essential as generators of interesting research questions. A precise and general understanding of how language is structured and functions is essential to the experimentalist's work, as much as a general understanding of the structure and function on any bodily organ or system, say the visual system, would be for the experimental study of the pathologies of the specific domain, vision or the like. In the absence of articulated models of mental computations for language, experimental approaches to language use, acquisition and pathologies run a very serious risk: an extraordinarily rich methodological apparatus, such as the one developed by modern experimental psychology, may end up being used to address relatively unsophisticated, unsystematic and narrow questions, questions stemming from mere common sense ideas about what language is and how it works, rather than from a sound scientific understanding emanating from fundamental research in the specific domain. Only well articulated and detailed models, endowed with a certain degree of deductive depth, embody hypotheses generating non trivial predictions, which may lead to significant empirical discoveries through the experimental testing.

From the viewpoint of theoretical linguistics, and the theory of syntax in particular, it is of fundamental importance to enlarge the empirical domains for testing hypotheses and models. Different empirical domains (say, language acquisition, the experimental study of production and comprehension, language pathology, brain imaging techniques applied to linguistic capacities) may provide critical evidence to choose between alternative hypotheses; converging evidence coming from different empirical areas and gathered through different techniques may offer a very robust kind of empirical support for particular formal ideas and models, reducing the risk of artifacts and potential methodological problems which may be linked to a single type of evidence. Moreover, the relation between theoretical modeling and experimental research should not be in just one direction (of the kind: models generate research predictions, and the experimental work tests them): clearly, there must be a feed-back effect such that the experimental results contribute to shape further research questions, and may directly suggests reformulations and refinements of the formal models; and reciprocally, particular questions generated by a formal model may contribute to shape new experimental methods well adapted to address them. So, the relationship between theory and experimentation must be dynamic and interactive, in language as in any other scientific domain.

Maria Garraffa's book provides a convincing illustration of how this interdisciplinary approach can shed light on the relationships between language structure and language pathologies. Garraffa's analysis combines precise grammatical hypotheses about syntactic structure-building, movement and locality, in the Principles and Parameters / Minimalist tradition, with structured hypotheses on the organization and functioning of the parser, as in the best tradition of theoretically informed experimental psycholinguistics, and with experimental techniques of elicited production, comprehension, and elicitation of metalinguistic judgments in an aphasic patient. The book offers a very rich picture of the spared and impaired syntactic capacities of the patient, thus contributing to a better understanding of the syndrome, and also providing insight on very general issues such as the relation between grammatical principles and the analytic strategies used by the human parsing system.

Luigi Rizzi
Siena, July 15, 2011

CHAPTER ONE

ACQUIRED LANGUAGE DISORDERS AND LINGUISTIC COMPUTATIONS

Introduction

In the theoretical linguistic model (Chomsky, 2000) the language faculty is defined as the manifestation of a particular cognitive faculty; a system of neural networks specified for linguistic computation. It is therefore reasonable to assume that the theoretical architecture of the linguistic model has a correlate in the organization of neural structures. According to this view, linguistic principles correspond to specific mental computations.

In this approach to language studies recent psycholinguistic investigations have integrated grammatical data with neurophysiological evidence to built spatial and temporal maps of the neural networks involved in language computation. Many studies of sentence processing have shown different effects according to the kind of information being parsed, from which assumptions can be drawn concerning the way the mind/brain deals with different linguistic information. For example, in Italian interesting evidence comes from reading time measures for processing of syntactic violations, such as subject-verb number agreement (as in: The beautiful baby *runs/run* in the garden) and semantic violations (e.g. selection features, as in: The trailhead *whistles/sprouts* at the station) (De Vincenzi et al., 2003). In the case of the syntactic violations, a delay on the verb followed by a quick return to the baseline was found. The semantic violations gave rise to an increase in reading time after the verb, which lasted until the end of the sentence.

More interestingly, a similar dissociation was shown using the EEG technique. Syntactic violations elicited an electrophysiological component in the left anterior areas in the 300-500 msec time frame, while semantic violations gave rise to a more central and later component, the so-called N400, a negative component.

This kind of evidences supports the view that there are distinct computations for different types of linguistic information: syntactic and semantic. Furthermore syntactic violations need to be repaired in a local interval, while semantic violations elicited a different measurable effect, with a non-clear index of a repairing procedure.

Many subsequent investigations have developed more finely-tuned models of language processing and linguistic theory could provide interesting means to define different linguistic computations.

The model elaborated by Angela Friederici (see Friederici, 2002 for an overview) is consistent with these types of evidence. In this model three temporally and spatially distinct phases of language comprehension are postulated: an early structural process subserved by the anterior part of the left hemisphere (as observed for categorial violations); a second, post-syntactic phase where lexical-semantic and argument structure are processed (with corresponding activation distributed over the left and the right temporo-parietal areas); and a process of structural reanalysis subserved by centro-parietal areas (as observed with brain imaging techniques).

There are divergent opinions on how these kinds of data are to be interpreted (see Osterhout, L., 2000; and Osterhout et al., 2009), and detailed cross-linguistic research is necessary.

A different empirical source supporting grammatical distinctions in the computation of linguistic information comes from the study of subjects with cerebral lesions.

Neurolinguistic observations are particularly interesting, providing the possibility of exploring specific properties of the linguistic faculty not manifested in normal speakers and evident in a non-fully-fledged cognitive system. In this field a notable step in integrating linguistic theory comes from study of the functional lexicon in the so-called agrammatic aphasia.

Friedmann and Grodzinsky (2000) proposed that in their patients the omission of items from the functional lexicon was sensitive to the position of these elements in syntactic structures. Starting from this original investigation, many cross-linguistic data have shown that not the entire functional lexicon is damaged in Broca's aphasia and more detailed investigation plausibly indicates the retrieval of closed class items in a grammatical structure (see chapter 1 of the present study).

For example, many cross-linguistic studies have shown a disassociation with respect to the omission of verbal inflection in the system: subject–verb agreement is preserved while temporal morphology is omitted.

Agreement and temporal dependencies are similar in the sense that both are related to feature matching. The agreement relation requires the number feature to be copied from the subject onto the verb, and in doing so establishes a configurational agreement relation. In temporal concordance a temporal adverb and the finite verb must share their tense feature.

In addition, the two grammatical dependencies have positional differences (these are well attested in the linguistic literature since Pollock's comparative studies on the Romance languages; Pollock, 1989). In the tree structure they occupy different syntactic phrases in a parameterized order. On the basis of this evidence, Friedmann developed the influential Tree Pruning Hypothesis. This is a pure representational account of grammatical disorders, and in our opinion a reflection on the source of the agrammatic syndrome is necessary.

A distinction between Tense and Agreement dependencies was also found in a recent study on processing in adult speakers (De Vincenzi, et al, 2010). In an ERP experiment on morphosyntactic feature matching, agreement violations were detected in an early phase while violations of temporal morphology were detected in a successive temporal window. This could be an indication of a sequential parsing model where purely formal syntactic operations, such as subject-verb agreement, precede post-syntactic analysis, such as the interpretation of incongruent temporal features.

This approach directly links evidence from language processing with evidence from linguistic theory. The different features comprising morphosyntactic information may be differently parsed both in temporal and in spatial terms, in line with theoretical evidence from linguistic models.

Differences in temporal and topographical patterns expressed in a model such as Friederici's, along with data from neuropsychology, are taken as evidence for the view that grammatical analyses are part of the parsing strategy, and grammatical options are parsing strategies.

In this sense, an aphasia such as the one studied in the present work may be explained as an impoverishment of the processing system.

The experiments presented here have been conceived to test grammatical properties as essential components of sentence processing. This shifts from the study of concrete constructions (such as passives, relatives, etc.) to more abstract computational operations (such as Movement, or Merge). To test the capacity of our subject to create a grammatical string, a configurational skeleton for the insertion of a contentive lexicon, we selected a series of well know theoretical phenomena involving syntactic factors.

The linguistic variables selected are mainly related to locality conditions in the sentence, implemented in a precise structural map as a rich cartographic set of tree positions (see Cinque G., 2002; Belletti A., 2004; Rizzi L., 2004).

The cartographic approach is a recent theoretical methodology codified to define a map of syntactic positions in tree structures. The fundamental idea behind this approach is that during the building of a syntactic sequence structural information is directly readable from the map. Not only is there a geometric constraint in the implementation of structural relations, other information, such as interpretative distinctions, is also structurally organized.

In the cartographic approach, neurolinguistic and psycholinguistic experiments showing dissociations between grammatical features, such as Tense and Agreement in aphasia or distinctions in the computation of different grammatical violations, could provide evidence for the presence of different structural positions in which different classes of grammatical features are implemented. Such experiments provide a rich source of evidence with which to corroborate linguistic theory.

Summary of findings

The experiments presented here have been conceived to test grammatical properties as essential components of sentence processing. This shift from the study of concrete constructions (such as passives, relatives, etc.) to more abstract computational operations (such as Movement, or Merge). To test the capacity of our subject to create a grammatical string, a configurational skeleton for the insertion of a contentive lexicon, we selected a series of well-known theoretical phenomena involving syntactic factors.

The linguistic variables selected are mainly related to locality conditions in the sentence, implemented in a precise structural map as a rich cartographic set of tree positions (see Cinque G., 2002; Belletti A., 2004; Rizzi L., 2004).

The cartographic approach is a recent theoretical methodology codified to define a map of syntactic positions in tree structures. The fundamental idea behind this approach is that during the building of a syntactic sequence structural information is directly readable from the map. Not only is there a geometric constraint in the implementation of structural relations, other information, such as interpretative distinctions, is also structurally organized.

In the cartographic approach, neurolinguistic and psycholinguistic experiments showing dissociations between grammatical features, such as Tense and Agreement in aphasia or distinctions in the computation of different grammatical violations, could provide evidence for the presence of different structural positions in which different classes of grammatical features are implemented. Such experiments provide a rich source of evidence with which to corroborate linguistic theory.

The results of various experiments run to investigate M.R.'s linguistic competence show selective impairment in object movement. The so-called canonicity effect has been attested since Caramazza and Zurif's seminal work (1976). Furthermore, in the present study a similar subject/object asymmetry emerges in interrogative sentence production, which has been found to be selectively impaired for object movement of animate arguments. This canonicity effect can be analyzed as a grammatical phenomenon (see Garraffa and Grillo, 2008). Structures resulting from movement, chains, obey certain locality principles, and may be subject to intervention effects due to the minimality condition (Rizzi, 1990; 2005). In a recent work, Grillo (2005) proposed that in agrammatic patients sets of features normally associated with syntactic heads can be underspecified where processing capacities are reduced, thus giving rise to selective minimality effects: structures where a dependency is constructed over an intervening DP are more problematic. Recent research on the processing cost of *crossing* relations vs. *nesting* supports this view (see for example Erdozia and Laka, 2009 for a study on agreement violations in Basque).

Furthermore, this impoverishment in the syntactic representation seems directly explainable in cartographic terms. In the cartographic approach, formal features (such as *WH*, or Discourse related features) are more prominent functional shells and they are represented in the upper periphery of the clause.

"Animacy" could be codified in a low tree position, close to the Noun lexical head. These features emerge in cases of grammatical impoverishment, such as in aphasia, and play a prominent role in the grammatical coding of the structure. Many studies on the role of animacy in processing have demonstrated rapid access to this kind of information (as an example see Kuperberg et al., 2006; Mak et al., 2002).

Such asymmetries are found in M.R.'s utterances, which show selective impairment of object movement for animate arguments, supporting the idea of a distinction in the grammatical implementation of features.

Normal syntactic representation

(1a) $_{CP/IP}$[+Wh, Nom, φsing, θ1,N,+Animacy] [+ Animacy] $_{VP}$[N,+Animacy]
Chi ***pro*** hai baciato < *Chi* > ?
Who *have[2°sing]kissed* < *Who* >?

Agrammatic syntactic representation

(1b) $_{CP}$[+ Animacy] [+ Animacy] $_{VP}$[+Animacy]
Chi ***pro*** hai baciato < *Chi* > ?
Who *have [2°sing] kissed* < *Who* >?

M.R.'s question production showed evidence of difficulties with object extraction in D-linked interrogative operators, such as "Quale" (*Which*). Copies of the noun phrase were found in situ in her speech, e.g. "*Quale libro hai letto un libro?*" (lit. Which book did you read a book?). This data is hardly explainable without the assumption that the deficit is of a grammatical nature.

An increase in processing cost attributed to the more subtle structural properties of extraction in sentences with a D-Linking operator is a well-attested phenomenon (see for example De Vincenzi, 1991, Rizzi, 2002 and Hickok and Avrutin, 1995).

These data on interrogatives may be interpreted as grammatical reduction of some of the formal features implemented in the syntactic tree. The result could be a reduced structure, *truncated* in Rizzi's sense.

(2)

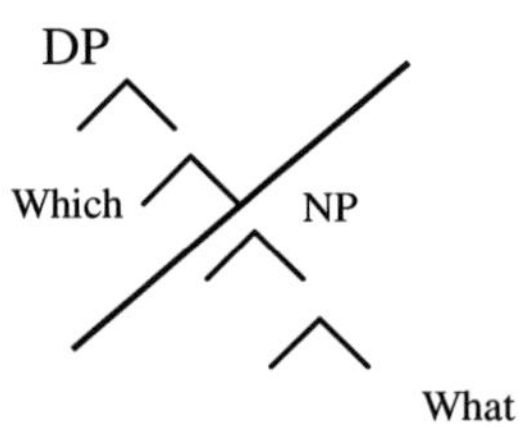

Interesting linguistic evidence, related to the syntax-semantic interface, that supports the present positional distinction comes from a study on the semantic properties of definiteness restriction (Heim, 1987). In her investigation on *Wh*-traces and definite variables Heim presents data related to "definiteness" of the moved *wh*-phrase, (example in (3) from Heim, ibidem pag. 27).

(3) a. ??Which one of the two men was there in the room/*drunk?
b. ??Which actors were there in the room/*laughing?
c. ?Who was there in the room when you got home?
d. What is there in Austin?

A sort of definiteness hierarchy seems related to the possibility of extraction of a Wh operator in "there is" constructions, with "What" the less specified operator and a licit extractable element. This fact could allow us to describe the non-standard linguistic competence of our patient: all extractions are treated as (3d), the one with the less specified operator.

Subsequently, we studied locality conditions in attraction configurations in a grammaticality judgment task. Much work in the psycholinguistic literature (e.g. Bock and Miller, 1991) shows that an intervening element, situated between the elements sharing an agreement relation, and mismatched in the relevant feature, attracts agreement, as expressed in the abstract configuration in (4).

(4) **X** **...** **Z** **...** **Y**
$[\ldots,\varphi_{Singular}]$ $[\ldots,\varphi_{Plural}]$ $[\ldots,\varphi_{Singular}]$

The boat of the American soldiers leaves in the fog
*The boat of the American soldiers leave in the fog

Attraction is readily explainable in terms of locality conditions and it offers a good testing ground for the proposal outlined here.

A recent study on the structural properties of agreement shows different effects in terms of different syntactic relations: linear precedence vs. hierarchical order (Franck et al. 2006). In this study, attraction effects with two different classes of interveners: prepositional modifiers (5a) and clitic object pronouns (5b) were investigated in French.

(5a) $[_{Subj} \ldots N_{head} \ldots \mathbf{N_{mod}} \ldots]$ AgrS
(5b) $[_{Subj} \ldots N_{head} \ldots]$ $[_{\mathbf{AgrOP}}$ **pro** $_{\mathbf{clitic}}]$ AgrS

The main finding of this experiment is significant numbers of attraction errors with clitics compared with prepositional modifiers. The authors explained this effect as a result of differences in the structural relations involved: in (5b) the intervening constituent, the clitic, is in a c-command relationship with the agreement head, whereas the prepositional modifier in (5a) is merely in a configuration of linear precedence. We investigated intervention in our case study with a grammatical judgment task, looking in particular at the different intervention effects in terms of their different structural relations, as in (6a) and (6b) (examples of the formalization expressed in 5).

(6a) [La nave dei soldati] parte/*partono nella nebbia
*[The boat of the soldiers] leaves/*leave in the fog*
(6b) Il corridore [li *inseguono/insegue]
*The runner [them *exceed/exceeds]*

M.R.'s responses show significant attraction effects caused by the intervention of a prepositional modifier, as in (6a). No effect was found with object clitics, as in (6b). A possible distinction in the nature of clitics emerges looking at cross-linguistic properties. In French clitics are weak pronouns, more independent elements than Italian clitics (in this sense see also Kayne on the possibility in French of positioning adverbs in between clitic and verb).

Crucially, no effect was found with normal Spanish speakers (Anton-Mendez, 1996) where object clitics are not active elements for agreement.

(7a) Las manzanas **las** he comid**o** [No Agr]
The apples them (pl) I have eaten
(7b) Le mele **le** ho mangiat**e**
The apples, them (f.pl.) I have eaten (f.pl.)

In processing term we attribute the absence of attraction effects with object clitics in this Italian aphasic speaker to non-computation of agreement relations in the object position, it being an intervener in the subject-verb relation.

The same explanation holds in both cases: the intervention of a clitic in the absence of a fully-fledged AgrO projection is not enough to induce minimality effects in Spanish speakers, nor in M.R.

The present approach on acquired language disorders makes precise predictions regarding the nature of the reduction in the procedural capacities and is compatible with parsing models that posit *on-line* construction of a syntactic representation during language production. The parser's preferences will be tied to both the structural characteristics of the sentence and to the predictions of the parsing principle.

An important aspect to the interpretation of our results in terms of a reduction of processing capacity was formalized in De Vincenzi's (1991) in a parsing strategy called *Minimal Chain Condition*:

MCC: Avoid postulating unnecessary chain members, but do not delay required chain members. (De Vincenzi, M., 1991)

We should expect limitations in forming chains over an intervening element where there is a reduction in the number (and quality) of features associated with each syntactic node. To test this prediction we investigate M.R.'s comprehension of relative clauses. The relevant variables of this study are word order and agreement mismatch between subject and object, allowing non-ambiguous interpretation. Non-standard word order, NP-NP-V, and Agreement mismatch force the grammatical system to build a syntactic chain to reach the correct interpretation. A clear impairment arises in non-canonical configurations.

The presence of a preverbal subject in the relative clause, as in *I ragazzi che il maestro ha salutato* (lit. The boys that il maestro has greeted), forces M.R. to revise her decision and the sentence is interpreted using agreement morphology.

Revision of a post-verbal subject in the relative clause, as in *I ragazzi che ha salutato il maestro* (lit. The boys that has greeted il maestro), takes place on the embedded verb. At this point material should probably be deleted for a limited memory source.

In the processing of obligatory filler-gap constructions (such as a relative clauses) the parser prefers to close the dependency and form a grammatical object: a syntactic chain. The differences between relatives with pre-verbal subjects and those with post-verbal subjects show the importance of making more finely-grained distinctions in the impaired system: differences in number features, which play a marginal role in normal language (probably due to the presence of higher order features) do, however, play a role in helping to cross a potential intervener in an impaired system.

The advantage of this approach is that it explains the way in which various elements are integrated in the syntactic structure. Furthermore, we can formulate precise predictions compatible with linguistic evidence. Systematic studies on features disambiguation involved in the grammar of languages could reveal interesting data for this investigation. This could underline different linguistic strategies for argument-marked languages and agreement-marked languages.

In the state of the art of language disorders a well-known and productive approach to agrammatism found a deficit in recognizing traces, a kind of empty position, in the linguistic string (Grodzinsky, 1990; 2000). According to this hypothesis, traces are deleted and their interpretations are not recoverable in the syntactic representation.

This approach to language impairment is not clear about how linguistic information is integrated in the structure, and consequently why traces should have a different nature. In Grodzinsky's system on agrammatic comprehension the interaction between an incomplete grammatical representation and a non-grammatical heuristic is established [NP1= Agent].

This heuristic is necessary in comprehension tasks, where the subject must assign thematic roles. The 'first agent' strategy applies only on NP's that have not received a thematic role by grammatical analysis. So a purely syntactic condition [-ϑ] selects the elements to which the strategy applies. In processing terms this means a syntactic analysis must first be made before the application domain of the strategy can be defined. Only after inconclusive thematic role assignment does the possibility of using this strategy arise.

An approach in terms of reduced information regarding a given grammatical principle and compatible with parsing strategies is more appropriate under the view that procedural capacity has a grammatical nature.

Furthermore, well-known problems such as cross-patient variability or the varying complexity of different syntactic strings are not difficult to overcome, since the processing costs could be structurally defined.

In sum, a neurological event can generate a reduction in the syntactic processing. This has visible and selective effects, verifiable by looking at the application of grammatical variables.

Crucially for the present approach, we observed impairment in comprehension and production of non-canonical structures due to the intervention of an extraneous element serving as a possible antecedent of the syntactic chain.

The fundamental spirit of this study is to account for the phenomena discussed in this case study, and possibly grammatical deficit in general, in terms of well-defined grammatical patterns.

CHAPTER TWO

CASE STUDY

M.R. is a 42-year-old right-handed Italian woman. She has aphasia caused by a focal lesion in the left hemisphere in frontal and parietal areas resulting from a stroke in the zone of the medial cerebral artery (MCA). The unilateral damage was ascertained by CT-scan. She was subjected to a clinical endovascular procedure.

After the lesion event the patient showed global aphasia and right hemiparesis. Her linguistic competence subsequently improved, until she reached a stage of non-fluent elliptical speech. Before the lesion event M.R. had worked as a doctor in an Italian hospital. She is aware of her linguistic deficit and was co-operative in the experimental sessions.

This study was conducted two years post-onset, by which time M.R.'s condition had stabilized.

Language screening was carried out with the standard battery for Italian speakers (B.A.D.A.) (Miceli et al., 1994). The most typical features which the screening revealed were: difficulties with object and action naming (43.3% of objects are correct, 57.1% of actions), non-fluent speech with omission of grammatical elements, an impairment in the comprehension of reversible sentences with inversion of thematic roles, failure in grammaticality judgments of object relative clauses (3/3) and of pronoun reference, and low scores in working memory tasks measured at word list level.

A selective impairment in the comprehension of reversible passives and object relative clauses and non-fluent speech with high omission of function words is generally classified as a grammatical impairment. Reading and writing abilities were also greatly impaired, but they will not be dealt with in this study.

1. Production

During the experimental sessions we collected a corpus of spontaneous speech production. M.R. has non-fluent speech and shows a deficit in functional words, such as copulas, auxiliaries, complementizers and determiners.

An example of her linguistic abilities in speech production is presented in the transcription reported below.

Recipe: The cream puff
… i bignè. Allora un uovo un un .Un? Burro.La..... acqua e.... Allora la la il tegamino. e mescola la …piano piano così
the cream puffs. Then an egg a a. A? Butter. The…water and…Then the the [sing,fem] the pan and mix the …gently gently like that
fin quando fin quando una pasta così così così. È bella. Poi poi mi mi … la tortiere.
till till a dough thus thus thus. Is good. Then then me me…the (sg.) cake tins.
Un pezzettino a un bignè un bignè un bignè al forno. Allora e cresce cresce ... il gas. Il gas no.
A little piece to a cream puff a cream puff a cream puff in oven.Then and grows grows… the gas.The gas no
Allora allora . forno forno. Poi questa qua pronta. Poi la ricotta. Io zucchero e il latte , il latte. E cuoce, no.
Then then. oven oven. Then this here ready. Then the ricotta. I sugar and the milk, the milk. And bake,no.
E poi piano piano …avvolgi avvolgi avvolgi e e mescola mescola mescola fin quando tutto.
And then gently gently… roll up roll up roll up and and mix mix mix till all.

M.R. is able to produce active declarative clauses.

However, in a constrained task she was not able to produce passive sentences. The task involved presentation of a picture illustrating an action, for example, the one described in (8); the experimenter points to the student in the picture in order to elicit the target sentence in (9).

Target:
(8) The student is greeted by the professor
M.R.'s production:
(9) The student greets the professor

In the next chapter we will investigate the functional lexicon in M.R.'s spontaneous speech production and will see that it contains many selective omissions.

2. Comprehension

The comprehension test of the standard battery B.A.D.A. is a picture-matching task. The items are semantically reversible sentences in active and passive voice. M.R. shows impairment with passives (12/17, 70.5% correct), yet made few errors with active reversible sentences (2/18, 11.1% incorrect). Moreover, in a grammaticality judgment task M.R. considered object relatives as non-grammatical sentences (3/3). We ran an extra battery of relative clauses and cleft sentences. Results are summarised in Table 1.

Sentence comprehension	**Correct**	**%**	**Sentences**
Subject cleft	18/20	90	E' il ragazzo che saluta il professore
Object cleft	8/20	40	E' il ragazzo che il prefessore saluta
Subject relatives	17/20	85	Il ragazzo che saluta il professore…
Object relatives	8/20	40	Il ragazzo che il professore saluta…
TOTAL	51/80	63.7	

Tab. 1 M.R.'s scores on sentence comprehension

These results show a selective deficit in the comprehension of reversible sentences with inversion of thematic roles.

To reach a better understanding of the patient's comprehension abilities an extra battery of object relatives was presented. Test items were object relatives with an agreement mismatch in the two arguments of the verb, e.g. *I ragazzi che hanno salutato il maestro* (The boys who have greeted the teacher).

We will discuss data on comprehension in more depth in chapter 6, where we also present other experiments on comprehension.

CHAPTER THREE

NOTES ON FUNCTIONAL ELEMENTS IN A CASE STUDY OF SPEECH: A STUDY ON VERBAL INFLECTION AND SUBJECT POSITIONS

Grammatical disorders are defined as non-fluent production characterized by a high omission rate of function words, low use of subordination and general use of short sentences.

More detailed analyses disclose that not all functional elements are impaired in agrammatic speech (Friedmann, 1998; and many related works). Based on the observation of selective omission of temporal morphology and preserved number feature in subject-verb agreement Friedmann has hypothesized a structural reduction of the syntactic tree (*The Tree Pruning Hypothesis*; Friedmann, ibidem).

In her view, this particular omission in verbal inflection could be an indication of specific selection driven by positional properties of the structure. In general, her hypothesis is that in agrammatic speech there is disturbed use of the functional architecture of the tree structure, an essential component of grammatical knowledge.

In this chapter we will describe some aspects of M.R.'s functional lexicon as evidenced in her spontaneous speech. M.R. shows an optional use of verbal morphology. She correctly produces number feature in subject-verb agreement relations, but she substitutes tense morphemes on verbs, as predicted by Friedmann's hypothesis. Furthermore, M.R.'s speech seems to be sensitive to certain related grammatical phenomena. Subject distribution (pre/post verbal and overt/null subjects) is selectively impaired and these phenomena seem to be related to a reduction in processing capacity. We will compare M.R.'s impairments as evidenced in her elliptical speech with the results from many studies on processing in adult systems. We propose that M.R.'s errors in spontaneous production represent an impoverishment of certain subtle syntactic distinctions and in reviewing the positional order of inflectional heads provide evidence in support of Friedman's idea of a structural reduction.

1. Notes on open/closed class items and lexical/functional heads

The elements that comprise the mental lexicon can be classified in two main categories: functional elements and contentive elements.

Functional elements form a closed class comprising lexical material such as determiners, auxiliaries, modals, copulas, conjunctions and complementizers. They are few and diachronically very stable (see Roberts 1993 for a study on the introduction of modals in English). They do not participate in derivational morphology and have "abstract" interpretative properties.

Contentive items form an open class of "descriptive contexts"; more properly they are lexical roots. They are not decomposed into grammatical features and are productive, participating in derivational morphology [1].

That the mental lexicon may be organized along these lines is made plausible by much evidence stemming from language acquisition, language use and pathology.

Psycholinguistic experimental studies of language use suggest that closed class items are accessed differently to open class items (Garrett; 1980). Research with Event Related Potentials (ERPs) suggests that distinct neural structures are involved in the access and use of elements of the two classes (Brown, Keurs and Hagoort, 1997; Neville, Mills and Lawson, 1992). Open class items elicit an electrophysiological negativity at 350msec (N350) in the posterior bilateral cerebral areas, considered a "signature" of a searching through the lexicon; closed class items elicit a negativity at 280msec (N280) localized in the left anterior temporal regions, a possible signature of grammatical selection. There are many more subtle aspects not encompassed in this classification. The distinction between open/closed items is too vague and does not capture certain

---

[1] Much research has refined the basic distinctions in the mental lexicon. An interesting suggestion comes from neuropsychological data on the distincion between Nouns and Verbs (see Caramazza and Shapiro, 2004). In their model, Nouns and Verbs may be selectivly damaged as they are represented by different neural networks.

These data are claimed to support a notion of the language faculty where specific neural networks correspond to specific linguistic descriptions (e.g. nouns could be the grammatical category associated with the cognitive representation of objects, verbs with the cognitive representation of events).

generalizations. For example, it would be interesting to investigate finer distinctions in the representations of homophones with different grammatical selection, such as clitics and determiners in Italian (e.g., *Lo* zaino 'The (m) rucksack', *lo* dimentico spesso in classe 'it I-forget often in class') or the difference between *to have* as an auxiliary, a functional word, and as a lexical verb, a contentive word.

In the early stages of language acquisition, around age 2, children typically use open class elements but omit closed class elements obligatory in their target grammar (see, for example, Chierchia and Guasti, 2000 for a study on determiners and Becker, 2000 for functional verbs). In early child language underspecification seems to be a widespread property of functional categories/features.

Much work on aphasia concerns the class of the functional lexicon, since the tendency to drop functional elements is characteristic of so-called agrammatic or non-fluent speech (see Menn and Obler, 1990 for an extensive cross-language overview). Slower recognition times for closed-class words than for open class words have been attested in many studies (see Friederici, 1995 for an overview). Broca's aphasics' recognition times for open class words are slower than normal speakers' times; the difference, however, was considerably less than that found with recognition of closed-class elements where Broca's aphasics' times were 250msecs lower than normal subjects.

Given this significantly slower recognition time with functional elements we wondered whether Broca's aphasics were able to access the structural information encoded in these elements. To investigate this question many experiments were run using different experimental paradigms. Interesting evidence emerged from the syntactic priming paradigm. In a study on German aphasics Friederici and Kilborn (1989) investigated access to the information carried by the auxiliary in sentences where grammaticality crucially depends on the combination of the auxiliary and the past participle, as in analytic verb forms (e.g., *Het meisje wordt geslagen* vs. *Het meisje wordt gereised*). The observed reaction time indicated that aphasics are able to access and use the information encoded in the closed class element. An interesting pattern that emerges from these studies is that Broca's aphasics' lexical decision times in sentence-based tasks were significantly slower (about 200-250 msec slower than the baseline measure) than in tasks with words in isolation. The reverse pattern was found for normal subjects: faster reaction times in sentence-based tasks compared with tasks where words were presented in isolation. These results support the hypothesis that a major aspect of grammatical deficit is related to the loss of automatic access and use of the syntactic information encoded in functional elements. Furthermore, these data are consistent with the approach proposed in this study and support the notion that parsing strategies are of an essentially grammatical nature.

The syntactic theory known as the Principles and Parameters framework (including more recent programs such as Minimalism) (e.g., Chomsky, 1995) posits that sentence computation involves the manipulation not only of lexical categories such as nouns and verbs, but also of functional categories. These largely correspond to function words, and, crucially, can also license inflection (e.g., tense, agreement). Therefore, a deficit in the syntactic manipulation of functional categories should impair not only function words, but also inflectional affixes (e.g., –*ed* in English) and non-affixed inflection (e.g., irregular past-tenses). Most importantly for our purposes, functional categories are concatenated stepwise into hierarchical structures, from subordinate (lower) to super-ordinate (higher) categories. Likewise, they trigger fundamental computations such as verb movement stepwise from subordinate to super-ordinate categories. An impairment of the operations of concatenation and/or movement should lower the likelihood of success of these operations. Because fewer of these operations are necessary to compute lower categories than higher ones, the lower the category, the easier it should be to compute.

In the literature on non-fluent agrammatic speech, it has been suggested that not the entire functional lexicon is necessarily damaged in aphasic patients, paving the way for finer distinctions to be made within this category.

An interesting find emerges from observation of selective omission of verbal inflection in agrammatic production. Friedmann's pioneering study on Hebrew and Arabic patients has drawn attention to an inconsistency in the omission of verbal morphology: in patients' spontaneous speech number agreement seems to be preserved while temporal morphology is highly impaired. Following Friedmann's study, much cross-linguistic empirical evidence has been gathered on dissociations in verbal morphology. The experiments have usually been run using a sentence completion task, such as the one presented below.

(10)Today the girl paints the room. Yesterday the girl _____ .
(11)Yesterday I jumped the fence. Yesterday they ________ .

Table 2 contains a summary of the cross-linguistic data from experiments on the split paradigm in verbal morphology using a sentence completion task.

Errors	Tense	Agreement	References
Hebrew (n=12)	42	4	Friedmann (1998)
Arabic(n=1)	69	9	Friedmann (1998)
Spanish (n=6)	94.5	36	Benedet et al. (1998)
English (n=7)	85	68	Christiansen and Goodglass (1998)
French (n=2)	Yes	No	Nespoulous et al.(1988)
German (n=7)	42	10	Wenzlaff and Clahsen (2004)
Spanish (n=7)	28.8	13.1	Gavarrò and Martinez (2003)
Catalan(n=7)	18	5.1	Gavarrò and Martinez (2003)
Galician (n=7)	41.7	8.8	Gavarrò and Martinez (2003)
Italian (n=1)	44.4	7.3	Garraffa (2010)

Table 2. Cross-linguistic studies on the Tense/Agreement distinction.

This cross-linguistic empirical evidence supports the idea that not the entire functional lexicon is impaired in agrammatic production. Grammatical deficit may instead be defined as a selective use of inflectional morphemes. The different distribution of Tense and Agreement supports the presence of a distinction in matching features in the inflectional domain. This could be interpreted as an indication of an active grammatical property in agrammatic production. Under this view, the morphology–syntax interface is considered a relation between functional features (syntax) and their exponents (morphology). These neuropsychological data provide a strong argument in favor of morphosyntactic features not being projected from overt morphology but instead being related to morphosyntactic variations. So, morphology has a partly realizational function: it interprets syntax.

Friedmann proposed linking the distinction in verbal inflection to a positional sensitivity related to different phrases in the syntactic tree.

Since Pollock (1989) much work in linguistic research has been directed towards a rich set of positions for the inflectional domain. Pollock's proposal, *The Split Inflection*, assumes that, at least in the Romance IP system, the features of finite verbal morphology play a crucial role. The most typical features are Tense and Agreement, the nature of Infl being more articulated. In the framework developed in Friedmann's proposal the positional distinction between Tense and Agreement follows a precise hierarchical order similar to the one proposed in Pollock's study: Tense>Agreement. The existence of a distinction between the lower (accessible) projections in the tree, such as those required for subject agreement and the more peripheral (inaccessible) positions in the syntactic representation of agrammatic speakers is the basis of the influential Tree

Pruning Hypothesis (Friedmann, 1998, 2002). In her view, selective impairment in agrammatic speech is caused by a reduction of the tree structure. This approach to functional omission provides a clear set of predictions upon which to base investigation of non-fluent speech. Furthermore, it posits that selection of grammatical items is related to syntactic structure.

In this chapter we look at the inflectional system, exploring M.R.'s production of agreement and tense morphology. We will address the issue of this optionality by looking at different subject positions as well as subject agreement in different syntactic domains: pre verbal and post verbal.

2. Inflectional morphology in M.R.'s productions: Tense and Agreement

This study is an examination of verbal morphology in M.R.'s spontaneous speech.

We collected her spontaneous speech for a period of four months composing a corpus of 132 narrative sentences. In the following tables some aspects of M.R.'s spontaneous speech are summarized. A common characteristic in non-fluent speech is the omission of functional elements. Table 3 shows M.R.'s low use of verbal functional elements in her spontaneous production.

Functional verbs N= 48	**Contexts**	**Productions**	**% omissions**
Auxiliaries	14	0	100
Copula	26	3	88.4
Lexical to have	8	2	75
TOTAL	48	5	89.5

Table 3. Distribution of verbal functional elements in M.R.'s spontaneous speech

Lexical verbs N= 84	Productions	Omissions
	60 (71.4%)	24 (28.6%)

Table 4. Lexical content verbs in M.R.'s spontaneous speech

An interesting aspect of M.R.'s production is the omission of lexical verbs. The data on lexical verbs, presented in table 4, demonstrates a different pattern of omission to that found with functional verbs. Lexical content verbs are non-standard but significantly less impaired than functional verbs.

Verbal morphology N= 60	Tense errors	Agreement errors
	21/60 (35%)	3/60 (5%)

Table 5. Tense and Agreement in M.R.'s sentence production

An analysis of M.R.'s spontaneous production of lexical verbs (60/84 items) shows a high percentage of substitution of Tense morphology but few errors in subject-verb agreement.

Similar data are attested in models such as Friedmann's Tree Pruning Hypothesis and are generally taken to be an indicator of a distinction between the two inflectional heads, Tense and Agreement. Moreover, it is interesting to note that the few agreement substitutions (3/60) are attested with post-verbal subjects. Of 18 verbs marked with plural number, 15 of their pre-verbal subjects are correctly inflected; in none of the VS plural forms is there subject-verb agreement. This does not constitute firm evidence but is nonetheless indication of a positional distinction in marking grammatical features.

Since data coming from spontaneous speech are quite variable (even if they are the most direct expression of linguistic competence), to test Friedmann's prediction on Split IP we ran a sentence completion task like the one used in the above-mentioned studies and exemplified in (10) and (11). In this task the subject must complete a sentence with the correct verbal form. The target response could be a temporal-inflected form or a number-inflected form.

Verbal morphology N=36	Tense errors	Agreement errors
	23/36 (63.8)	2/36 (5%)

Table 6. Tense and Agreement in a sentence completion task

Table 6 reflects the distinction between Tense and Agreement as reported in many cross-linguistic studies (see Table 2). As we have argued, this could be considered a sign of active grammatical properties in M.R.'s competence.

Friedmann's explanation of the Split IP dissociation is directly linked to the argument postulated in Pollock's study and to the idea that the Tense phrase (TP) occupies a position above the Agreement phrase (AgrP). On the other hand, many cross-linguistic data and evidence from generative syntax and from acquisition data are in favor of a subject agreement head higher than the Tense node (see Belletti, 2000 and Guasti and Rizzi, 2002 for a complete discussion)[2].

Furthermore, in our approach grammatical underspecification (as a selective impairment in verbal morphology) has to be explainable in terms of processing preferences, since our assumption is that grammatical selection is a parsing strategy. In a case study of an aphasic patient this kind of procedural explanation is also more suitable since it indicates the source of the deficit.

Interesting evidence in support of this view comes from a recent study on processing in adults (De Vincenzi et al., 2010). In this research reading times and event-related potentials were collected to investigate the parser's response to morphosyntactic violations: number violations and tense violations on verbs. In essence, this study is an investigation of the parsing processes of the Split IP. They studied subject-verb agreement and adverb–verb concordance, two local dependencies. Both relations involve an adjacent feature-matching operation and are established in a local configuration: in a Spec/Head structural relation as in (12) and (13).

[2] Other adult systems provide evidence in favour of a dissociation of the two positions. In certain languages it appears that Agreement is responsible for assigning case: Portuguese infinitives (+ Agr, - T) may be nominative case-marked; while in Belfast English case is not assigned to the subject of a tensed verb (- Agr, + T).

(12)

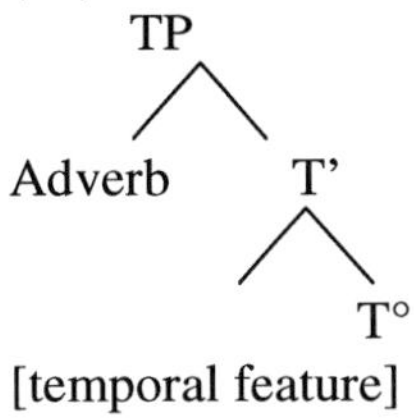

(13)

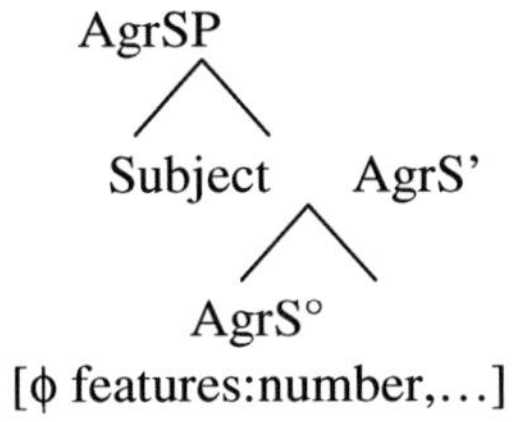

On the other hand, the two relations differ in the quality of features implemented.

In recent linguistic models (see Chomsky, 2000 for a detailed formal explanation) an important distinction is made between different types of features. In these approaches, they are divided into two main classes: interpretable features and uninterpretable features. Chomsky's model assumes that uninterpretable features enter the derivation unvalued. They must be assigned a value by a formal operation, Agree, and then deleted from the syntax.

Subject-verb agreement is an asymmetric relation: the number feature is interpretable on the subject and formally uninterpretable on the verb, needing to be assigned a value on the verbal head. In simpler terms, the number feature expressed on the noun predicates the singularity or the plurality of the referent. Number on the verb is a copied feature that has to be assigned a value for formal reasons. So, number on the verb is uninterpretable and needs to be assigned a value in a proper structural environment: a Spec/Head configuration.

Temporal features are interpretable in both elements: adverbs and verbs. The two features are independent (there can be temporal adverbs and verbs without temporal adverbs). Their concordance is interpreted at the post-syntactic level.

Distinctions in the implementation of Agreement and Tense features are predicted by generative syntax. (12) and (13) have the same structural configuration yet involve two different matching operations: the copying of features (subject-verb agreement) and the concordance of two interpretable features (adverb-verb agreement). The first is a purely syntactic process, while the latter involves a semantic representation and takes place at the post-syntactic level. In the above-mentioned study (De Vincenzi, et al, ibidem) different reading times and ERP responses were found for the two violations. Number violations in subject-verb agreement elicited a left anterior negativity (LAN) 60 msec earlier than the LAN elicited by Tense concord. Furthermore, in temporal violations the negativity is located in the right hemisphere.

Two points fall out from these data on the adult system. . Firstly, the evidence is consistent with models that make a distinction between syntactic and semantic processes, with distinct temporal phases (as in Friederici's model; see Friederici (2002) for a review).

Secondly, there is converging evidence (from behavioral, electrophysiological and neuropsychological data) for a distinct processing of the two morphosyntactic relations.

Data from cases of cerebral lesion, such as in the cross-linguistic studies summarized in Table 1 and that of the present study, complement the evidence from normal adult systems. Furthermore, the evidence opens up discussion on the possible source of grammatical impairment in neuropsychology: a pure *knowledge-based* argument, such as the one advanced in Friedmann's Structural Tree Pruning hypothesis, related to positional variables, or a more integrated approach in which grammatical distinctions are processing aids in parsing sentences. Speculation on these approaches to the language faculty requires examination of more finely-detailed grammatical phenomena and for grammatical selection to be investigated using psycholinguistic methods. In the next paragraph we will present other data collected from M.R.'s production and compare them with evidence from psycholinguistic studies.

3. Subject-Verb agreement and subject positions

In this paragraph we look at the relation between subject-verb agreement and subject position. The relevant variable investigated is the interplay between two possible subject orders, pre-verbal and post-verbal, and the morphological realization of agreement. Before presenting the data we will sketch some basic properties of the Italian grammatical system (see Belletti 2000 for further details). Italian is a null subject language with a rich morphological system. The standard word order is SVO, but a VS order is also allowed, as in (14c).

(14) a. In genere Maria ordina per tutti
Normally Maria orders for everybody
b. In genere *pro* ordina per tutti
Normally *pro she*-orders for everybody
c. In genere ordina Maria per tutti
Normally orders Maria for everybody
Maria normally orders for everybody

This free order is common in many null subject languages. VS order is also possible in non-null subject languages, but restricted to specific verbal classes (unaccusative verbs) as in (15). Italian is not subject to this restriction, VS order being possible with all verb classes, as in (16).

(15) a. There come three girls
b. Trois filles sont arrivées
three girls have arrived
c. Il est arrivé trois filles
it has arrived three girls
d. Sono arrivate tre ragazze
they-are arrived three girls
Three girls have arrived

(16) a. E' arrivata Maria.
has arrived Maria
Maria has arrived
b. Ha parlato Maria
has spoken Maria
Maria has spoken
c. Lo ha comprato Maria
it has bought Maria
Maria has bought it

Otherwise, there are specific conversional contexts eliciting a post-verbal subject. For example, the expected answer to a question such as (17) is (17b), with VS order. This preference is pragmatically determined. It is possible to have a preverbal subject only if focused, as in (17c). Data of this type are important for understanding the link between syntax and the informational context of the sentence[3].

(17) Quando sei entrato chi cantava?
When did you arrived who was singing?
a.*Maria cantava
b. Cantava Maria
c. MARIA cantava (non Lucia)

---

[3] This kind of evidence is the object of more fine-grained research in the cartographic approach to structure. The basic intuition on this approach to structure is that a specific intepretation is directly readable from the position of the elements comprising the sentence. In this way the intepretative system can read the cartographic map and reach the correct intepretation.

An interesting property of VS order is the difference in realization of agreement morphology. (15) illustrates that in English and French there are two possibilities[4]. English realizes morphological agreement as in (15a), whereas in French the post-verbal subject does not agree with the verb (15b vs. 15c).

In this paradigm standard Italian patterns with English (compare 6d with 6a) while some Italian dialects pattern with French (data reported in 18 are from Brandi and Cordin, 1989):

(18) Fiorentino / Florentine dialect

a. Gl'è venuto le su' sorelle
   to-him is come the his sisters

b. Le su' sorelle le son venute
   the his sisters they are come

Trentino/ Trentino dialect

c. E' vegnù le so' sorele
   is come the his sisters

d. Le so' sorele le son vegnude
   the his sisters they are come

This positional effect is also found in the acquisition literature (data form Rizzi and Guasti; *ibidem*). English 3-year-olds show a distinction between negative *do* and interrogative *do*. Typically, English children first produce negative sentences with uninflected *do*; these forms then alternate with the inflected ones and subsequently disappear.

(19) a. Robin don't play (Adam28, 3;4)
     b. so Paul doesn't wake up (Adam28, 3;4)

This optionality in inflection is virtually absent in interrogative contexts, as in (20).

(20) a. *Do he go?
     b. Does he write? (Adam28, 3:4)

---

[4] This argument is based on Rizzi and Guasti 2002; we refer the reader to this article for an exhaustive analysis.

These observations are consistent with the idea that realization of agreement is related to the positional properties of the elements concerned and support a grammatical interpretation of the phenomenon.

Guasti and Rizzi (ibidem) suggested an explanation for this morphosyntactic distinction in terms of different configurations. In SV structures agreement is checked twice: AgrS gets valued through AGREE, and its features are then checked, after movement of the subject, in a local Spec/head configuration. In VS structures agreement is established only under AGREE, as agreement checking in the local Spec/head configuration is not available. The two configurations are exemplified in (21).

(21) DP…AGR → syntactic checking
AGR…DP → specific property of the system

As seen in 15c and in 18, in post-verbal configurations morphological realization of number is not mandatory.

Since different agreement realizations can be considered in terms of fluctuation of the grammatical system we have a precise framework in which to evaluate M.R.'s performance on post-verbal subject agreement. For the present purposes, it is important to study different agreement configurations and to consider the performance of a non-fluent Italian speaker within this framework.

In a corpus of 60 sentences with verbs, M.R. produced 10 post-verbal subjects. No pre-verbal subjects were produced in contexts requiring a post-verbal subject. Subject distribution in M.R.'s production is summarized in Table 7.

	SV	VS	Total
Transitive	13	2	33
Unergative	12	1	13
Unaccusative	7	7	14
Total	32	10	60

Table 7. Distribution of subjects in M.R.'s spontaneous speech

In List A we report M.R.'s utterances in which the subject is in post-verbal position. Missing elements are written below each sentence.

LIST A

1	ed ecco	venuto io Maria Teresa e Gino.
	and there	came (p.p.) I Maria Teresa and Gino
	SIAMO VENUTI	
	we-are come	*(we came)*
2	Dopo	a trovare io
	after	to find I
	LE VADO	
	to-her go *(1st.p.)*	
3	Dieci giorni	riporta io Chiara, marito
	ten days	brings-back I Chiara, husband
	DOPO	MIO MARITO HA RIPORTATO ME E
	later	my husband has brought-back me and ...
4	Bussa la porta # un	principe # la scarpetta d'oro
	he-knocks the door #	a prince # the little-shoe of gold
	CON	
	with	
5	Lavorare tu?	
	to-work you?	
	TU LAVORI?	
	you work?	
6	e dopo	andato a Sonnino io Gino,
	and after	gone to Sonnino I Gino
	SIAMO ANDATI	
	we-are gone	(*we went*)
7	un anno	vissuto io
	a year	lived (*p.p.*) I
	HO	
	I-have	
8	parte figlio piccolo … nonna	
	leaves son little .....grandma	
	MIO CON LA	
	my with the	
9	arrivo dopo pranzo… ospedale	
	I-arrive after lunch ... hosital	
	E' ARRIVATO IN	
	is arrived in	
10	Sale la zia nella casa	
	goes-up the aunt in-the house	
	SALI'	
	went-up	

List A. M.R.'s utterances featuring post-verbal subjects.

In VS sentences the marked form of number agreement, plural morphology, is not produced (see utterances 1, 6 and 8).

It is interesting to note (in utterances 3 and 4) a VOS order as a possible consequence of lack of movement of the object phrase. This is clearly manifested in the absence of a case marker (as in 3) and in the presence of an indefinite NP in a context requiring a definite one (as in 4). A definite NP is an NPs whose Spec is filled by a definite article or a proper name.

In the VS utterances presented in List A Tense is underspecified, giving rise to non-finite forms. These utterances show underspecification of Tense and Agreement. This may indicate a structural distinction in agreement positions. In the previous paragraph we reported a well-established generalization on preserved Agreement features in SV order (see Table 2 and M.R.'s data). Friedmann (1998, 2002, and other works) has pointed out possible configurational effects and explained them in term of pruned phrase structures. In these VS utterances we see no Agreement features (nor case markers) and no Tense features. A possible representation in terms of tree positions is posited below.

(22)

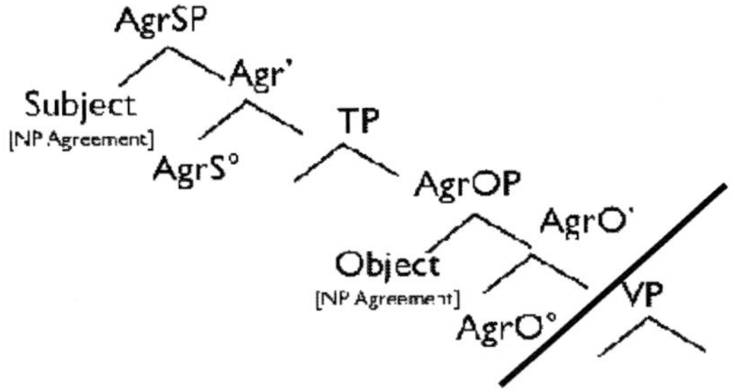

A direct consequence of this assumption is that in this case study subject agreement could be checked in a local configuration in an Agreement phrase not specified for object/subject, such as a low agreement position, probably the head for non-finite verb forms, AgrPstPSrt in a model compatible with much linguistic evidence (see Belletti,2000)[5].

---

[5] This possibile view is also supported by M.R.'s correct performance on participle agreement (80%). In Italian, participle verbal forms have to agree in gender and number with a noun object or subject, depending on the specific configuration. Generally the verb has to reach the relevant head for checking agreement features, AgrPstPart. M.R. productions are not standard, lacking auxiliaries. Otherwise

(23)

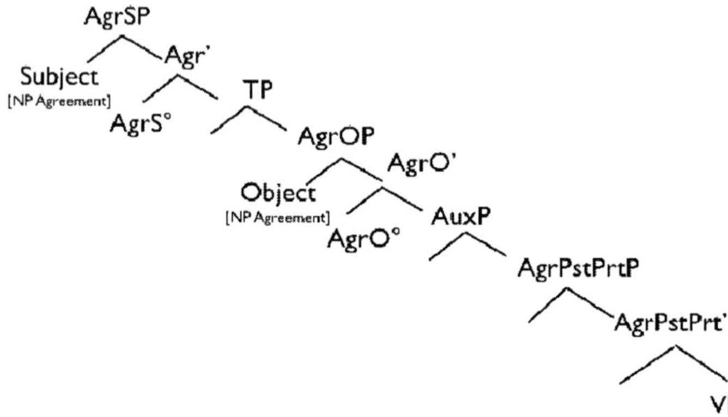

(Belletti, 2000)

These data allow us draw some more general assumptions. In a tree structure such as the one exemplified in (23) Tense seems to be the relevant node to distinguish between AgrS and AgrO. More generally, an Agreement node could be a maximal projection of a sentence or of a noun phrase. The distinction between the nodes is the consequence of different outcomes for incorporation of the head. An Agr combined with a Tense necessarily corresponds to a sentence representation and is compatible with selection by a complementizer. The consequence is that if we have a fully-specified Tense node we have a CP argument; the other possibility is a DP argument.

If Tense is not fully specified in aphasics' utterances the syntactic information is not enough to distinguish between a C- argument and a D-argument, i.e. between a sentence and a noun. A possible outcome of this speculation is the presence of nominalizations in verbal contexts rather than nominal ones. As is well attested, this is another typical feature of agrammatic productions (see Menn and Obler, 1990 for cross-linguistic data). This tentative explanation of the deficit needs to be tested with more data containing the relevant structures; for the moment we limit ourselves to speculation on the reduced structures.

---

agreement features are correctly marked. The evidence of gender and number features in these productions could be interpreted as a sign of a relation between participle form and the nominal subject in a low agreement position. A correct performance on Past Participle agreement was also reported in another study on two Italian subjects (De Bleser and Luzzatti, 1994).

From the argument just developed, a possible explanation of M.R.'s spontaneous speech is that it is shows a reduced structure and selective use of a low agreement position, AgrPstPrt, to check agreement of the external argument. This position is specific to non-finite constructions and it does not check other relevant syntactic features as other agreement positions do (AgrSP, AgrOP).

As an interim conclusion, we can state that M.R.'s production data are consistent with impoverishment of grammatical features. This impoverishment is reflected in a reduced tree structure compatible with structural grammatical selection, and a selective preference for low tree positions.

4. Eliciting post-verbal subjects

Since subject positions (more properly, non-local agreement checking) seem a possible variable to investigate the status of agreement relations, we ran a test specifically designed to elicit production of post-verbal subjects. The experiment is a picture-constrained production task. The task was originally created to test L2 acquisition of specific properties of Italian grammar, such as the possibility of placing a subject post-verbally. The task was designed for second language speakers with near-native competence in Italian (see Bennati, Belletti and Sorace, 2007). It consists of the elicitation of answers to questions whose pragmatic contexts require a response with a post-verbal subject (24). Test items were randomized and presented with filler sentences eliciting pre-verbal subjects, as in 25. Examples of test and filler items are presented below.

(24) Context requiring a post-verbal subject:
Chi è arrivato?
Who is arrived?
Target:
E' arrivato un ragazzo.
Is arrived a boy.

(25) Context requiring a pre-verbal subject:
Cosa fa il cameriere?
What is the waiter doing?
Target:
(Il cameriere) stappa la bottiglia.
The waiter is uncorking the bottle.

Test items eliciting post-verbal subjects were equally divided between unergative and unaccusative verbs.

The task was to produce a full verbal sentence. In fact, in Italian a simple noun or a null subject sentence would be a possible answer. M.R. showed no difficulties in carrying out the task. Of over 40 contexts eliciting a post-verbal subject M.R. produced 23 VS sentences. Many unaccusative verbs displayed a VS order (18/24). The data are summarized in Table 8.

	Unaccusative	Unergative	Total
SV	6/24 25%	11/16 69%	17/40
VS	18/24 75%	5/16 31%	23/40

Table 8. M.R.'s elicited production of post-verbal subjects

M.R.'s performance on this task resulted in two interesting findings. First, M.R. manifests a preference for VS order with unaccusative verbs (75%). Second, this preference seems related to the verb class. A post-verbal subject is not preferred with unergative verbs (31%).

As illustrated in (14), in Italian VS order is not sensitive to verb class, since we can have post-verbal subjects with all verb classes. However, in this experiment we obtained different results with unaccusative and unergative verbs. An interesting observation related to this data is presented in a study on first language acquisition (Lorusso, 2003; Lorusso et al., 2005 and Garraffa and Lorusso, 2007). In Lorusso's longitudinal study of the speech of 4 children aged between 18 to 39 months subjects use is sensitive to the type of verbs. It is greater with unaccusative than unergative verbs, a phenomenon that is also observed in the input. These results are evidence that children's syntactic representations of sentences with unaccusative and with unergative verbs are distinct and they may also suggest a preference for the ergative pattern in early language.

Data on caregivers showed that the SV order was preferred in declarative utterances with "transitive" and "unergative" verbs but not with unaccusative verbs. In this case, high frequency of VS order is predicted by the hypothesis that the subject is generated in the position of the internal argument and remains there, where it is likely to accomplish a different discourse-related function from a preverbal subject.

A possible explanation may lie in the different configurations involved in thematic assignment in the two verb classes. Several linguistic analyses assume a direct thematic role assignment for the subject of unaccusative verbs. Under this view the subject of unaccusative verb is a surface direct object.

(26)

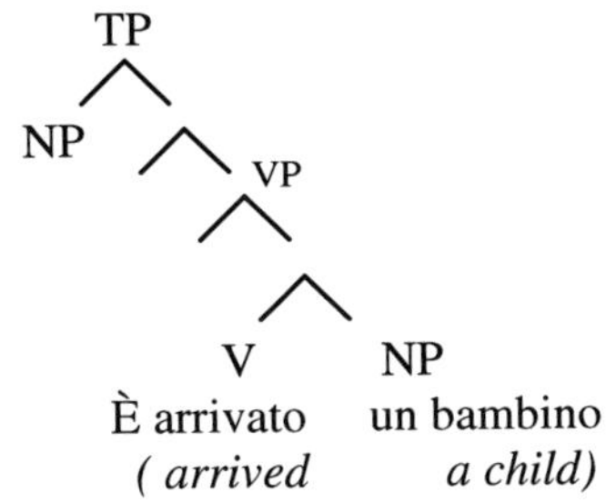

(27)

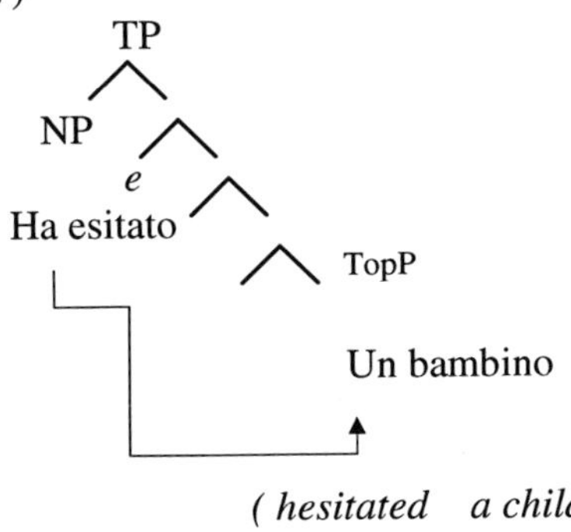

As exemplified in (26) and (27), only unergative verbs need to establish a dependency in order to link the two positions for assignment of the thematic role. With unaccusatives chain formation is not required and the grammatical subject in object position does not share any pronominal feature with the preverbal subject position.

(28) a. *pro* è arrivata Maria
b. pro_i ha esitato $Maria_i$

The two different configurations have been tested in sentence parsing (De Vincenzi, 1991). De Vicenzi's study tested adults' reading times on declarative sentences with post-verbal subjects. The experiment showed that VS structures with unaccusative verbs were easier to process than ones containing unergatives. This evidence strongly supports the hypothesis that chain formation is a costly process for the human sentence parser. Furthermore, a different pattern emerges with null subjects: both verb classes show slower reaction times with null subjects than with overt subjects, as they involve the licensing of a null category.

In his extensive research on Italian, De Vincenzi proposed a general heuristic pervading syntactic structure, *The Minimal Chain Condition (MCC)*[6]. Basically, he argues that if the parser has a choice in the derivation of a structure it prefers shorter chains. The principle is formalized in (29).

(29) *MCC: Avoid postulating unnecessary chain members, but do not delay required chain members.*

A chain is a set of coindexed elements (or positions) bearing one Theta-role and one case. To form a chain, this set of elements must respect configurational requirements (locality, c-command). A formal description of this syntactic object is presented in (30).

(30) Formal definition of chain:
$(A_1, \ldots A_n)$ is a chain if $1 <= i < n$:
$A_i = A_i+1$ [identity principle]
A_i c-command A_i+1 [prominence]
A_i+1 is in Minimal Configuration with A_i [locality]
(Rizzi, 1990)

Paraphrasing (30), a chain has to contain two elements of the same class (identity principle); one must be in an antecedent position (for example a c-command domain) and the empty element must be governed by the nearest antecedent (locality condition).

The second part of the MCC can be translated into another parsing principle elaborated by Frazier (1989), *The Active Filler Hypothesis.*

(31) Active Filler Hypothesis: *Once an element of the category XP is identified as moved from its argument position, then posit a corresponding empty XP category as soon as the grammar of the language allows you to do so. In this case posit the shortest chain at any given argument position.*

---

[6] We will mention this principle again in chapter 5 regarding a similar preference found in a comprehension task on post-verbal subjects in relative clauses.

We will analyze these two principles in depth and their possible connection with a grammatical explanation in chapters 5 and 6. For the purpose of this chapter suffice it to note that grammatical preference is related to preferred parsing strategies. This convergence of evidence supports our view that the linguistic parser is intrinsically grammatical in nature.

Furthermore, in M.R.'s utterances there are agreement errors which may be related to the subject position: 5 mistakes in VS order were found. This confirms her tendency to have agreement violations in VS order only with plural items, as in 32.

(32) Scende dal treno due ragazzi. (M.R.)
Get (sing.) off the train two boys

Our case study speaker seems to have a selective problem in realizing agreement in VS configurations, that is, non-local feature checking. Furthermore, the task on subjects in VS sentences shows that her competence on post-verbal positions with unaccusative verbs is good. This is important, as it allows us to exclude possible independent effects related to VS order *per se.*

M.R.'s preference for the post-verbal position with unaccusative verbs could be attributed to differences in the syntactic relations involved in checking subjects and to a preference on the part of the parser for a less costly operation.

5. Overt/null subject distribution and verb classes

In this section we will present data on the distribution of grammatical subjects in relation to verb classes in M.R.'s utterances. We looked at subject positions and *pro drop*, where agreement plays an important role in identifying the content of the empty category. Subject phrases in M.R.'s spontaneous speech do not seem to have the same distribution for the various verb classes. The DPs generated in a VP internal position are less likely to be omitted than DPs generated in an external position. Furthermore, the former are more likely to be expressed in post-verbal position than the latter.

We found that all null subjects occurred with transitive verbs.

	SV	VS	*pro* V	Total
Transitive	13	2	18	33
Unergative	12	(1)	-	13
Unaccusative	7	7	-	14
Total	32	10	18	60

Table 9. Distribution of subjects in M.R.'s spontaneous speech

Another study with a Hebrew aphasic speaker (Friedmann, 2000) showed a similar pattern in a repetition task: illicit *pro* drop occurred mainly with transitive verbs 64% (9/14); *pro* drop with intransitive verbs is relatively rare 6% (1/15)[7]. In these utterances case must be checked grammatically, and *pro* is also illicit for agrammatics.

Hebrew is only a partial null subject language. It is generally assumed that a rich agreement system plays a crucial role in the licensing of null subjects. Indeed, the distribution of *pro* varies across tenses and across persons. The complex distribution of NS in Hebrew is related to an agreement which is rich enough to be able to license the feature specification and the syntactic category of the empty element. Specifically, null subjects are licit when the category and feature specification of agreement matches the category and specification of the null pronoun. So, present Tense is unspecified for person and is not capable of identifying a reference for a null subject.

An interesting proposal regarding the role of inflection in licensing the position of *pro* in Hebrew and in VSO languages such as Irish, Welsh and Chamorro is presented in Doron (1988).

The author presents data in support of the claim that null subjects in Hebrew are licit only when the pronoun is in a 'clitic configuration', a particular configuration where the features of the complement are all contained in the features of the head.

In a clitic configuration Case is assigned to the clitic on the head and thus the features of the head, and not of the complement, are phonetically realized.

In the case study reported in Friedmann, subject pronouns were missing in contexts not licit for *pro* in standard Hebrew: third person tensed sentences.

An interesting aspect of her data is the correlation between the omission of subject pronouns and the argument properties of verbs: a low

[7] It is relevant for this study that the task involves only third person pronouns and that in Hebrew pro drop is not licit in this environment.

rate of subject pronouns is found with transitive verbs (5/14, 36%) in comparison with the repetition of subject pronouns with intransitives (14/15).

In addition, subject omission with this patient occurs with Tense substitutions and not only with the use of finite forms in matrix sentences.

A possible suggestion is that transitive verbs have a more complex thematic representation and they are more prone to errors. This suggestion is in line with Lorusso's data.

The performance of the patient is thus attributable to the same explanation: avoidance of more complex configurations results in a preference for null subjects with transitive verbs.

In this chapter we have presented an extensive analysis of M.R.'s spontaneous speech production. In her speech we found many indications of sensitivity to grammatical properties. The data collected point to a preference for grammatical constructions requiring less processing cost. To support our assumptions, we presented psycholinguistic evidence related to the findings reported in M.R.'s utterances. The main conclusion of this extensive analysis of M.R.'s speech is that her linguistic ability can be explained in terms of the grammatical framework discussed here and her speech is consistent with certain grammatical restrictions.

We introduced a parsing strategy compatible with the data collected in this case study, assuming non-preference for chain formation, as this involves more processing cost. This approach appears to be amenable to the investigation of the grammatical aspects of sentence processing.

CHAPTER FOUR

LINEAR AND HIERARCHIC RELATIONS: A STUDY ON INTERVENTION

In this chapter we investigate morphosyntactic properties of Subject-Verb (S-V) agreement. In order to analyze agreement relations in M.R.'s grammatical competence in depth we manipulated the position of constituents in an experiment on pre-verbal and post-verbal subjects. We also tested the occurrence of agreement errors in an attraction configuration, comparing linear vs. hierarchical order. This experiment involved grammaticality judgments on SV and VS agreement relations with different categories of interveners (prepositional modifiers and object clitics). Two phenomena in particular were analyzed: morphological realization of agreement in sentences with the subject in post-verbal position, and attraction effects on agreement between subject and verb in a task involving agreement mismatching in sentences with interveners such as: *La barca dei soldati americani è veloce*, (lit."The boat (f.sg.) of the soldiers (m.pl.) American is fast").

The patient showed difficulty in computing agreement features with post-verbal subjects. Furthermore, attraction effects are not manifested with post-verbal subjects, suggesting linear computation of the agreement relation.

Regarding attraction, M.R. does not show any interference in a grammatical judgment task in sentences with clitic interveners between subject and verb, as in *La professoressa le scrive* (lit."The teacher them writes"). On the other hand, she is highly sensitive to the interference of a prepositional modifier.

The main finding of this study is a selective impoverishment of agreement features related to the syntactic configuration in which agreement relations are implemented. We propose an explanation of this phenomenon in terms of minimality effects related to impoverishment of features in non-local syntactic configurations.

A cross-linguistic comparison with adult speakers shows similar effects in Romance languages where object clitics more strongly disrupt agreement relations in French than Italian and Spanish.

1. The study

In this chapter we take a further look at this selective impoverishment in the inflectional domain by investigating M.R.'s ability to perceive agreement violations. As mentioned in Chapter 3, M.R. correctly shows subject-verb agreement. Good performance on agreement morphology is also well-attested cross-linguistically (see chapter 3 for a detailed discussion).

In addition, we checked her production on different agreement configurations, and found a possible deficit in agreement inflection related to the subject position. It seems that agreement with post-verbal subjects is more likely to be omitted.

To test morphosyntactic agreement we manipulated two possible syntactic variables: position of constituents (post-verbal subjects) and the syntactic relation of a potential intervener in attraction configurations (linear precedence vs. c-command). We created a battery of grammaticality judgment tasks including agreement errors induced by the variables selected.

In this experiment we wanted to test two orders of grammatical relations:

a. agreement implemented via Agree without a Spec/X° configuration (as in VS order);

b. intervention effects in different attraction configurations (linear order configurations and hierarchical order, prepositional modifiers and object clitics).

Under the view that agreement processes can be taken to be the reflex of an established Spec/head relation inside an Agr projection, as revealed by (pre-verbal) subject agreement, post-verbal subject position agreement involves checking in a non-local configuration, and the building of a syntactic chain.

Concerning the research question expressed in b., intervention effects are related to the feature geometry that composes the structure. Furthermore, since intervention in attraction configurations is readily explainable in terms of minimality, even in the absence of c-command, it offers a testing ground to study agreement and locality effects.

2. Notes on subject agreement

Agreement is a morphosyntactic operation. It governs grammatical functions such as case assignment and Subject-Verb predication. In the standard theory of agreement two computational operations are the essential components of this relation: AGREE and MOVE. The former involves a probe and a goal. A probe conducts a search in its c-domain (sister node) to find a possible goal. MOVE is the verification of grammatical features (such as person and number) in specific positions: a local Spec/head configuration, for example, in an AgrSubject phrase (AgrSP). In this phrase the specifier hosts the subject and the head hosts the verb to establish a local relation. A possible tree representation is shown in (33) (see Belletti 2000 for an extensive discussion).

(33)

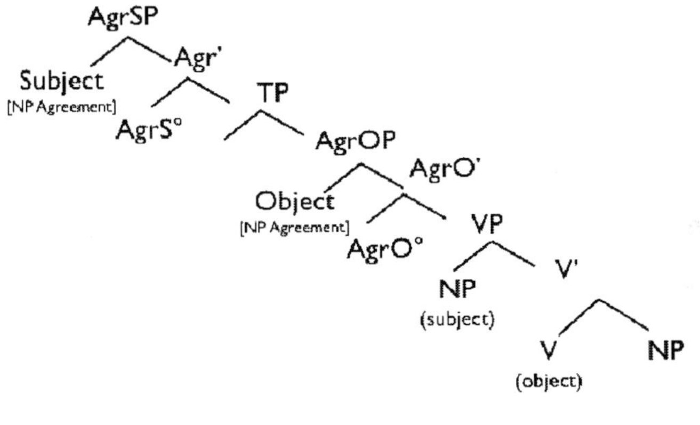

In this approach, as presented in chapter 3, the morphosyntactic interface is considered a maximally transparent relation: distinct positions in the structure (functional heads) license distinct morphosyntactic features. Agreement is thus manifested in a strict association between form and position.

As observed in chapter 3, the study of subject positions shows that morphological realization is dependent upon whether a feature has been checked in the overt syntax or not.

(34a) DP...Agr → configurational syntactic checking
(34b) Agr...DP → non-configurational syntactic checking

The formalism expressed in (34) presents Agreement as a grammatical process related to hierarchical factors. We will see that at a processing level this effect is visible and in configurations such as (34b) the system is more prone to error (agreement has variable morphological expression).

The agreement case studied here is Subject-Verb predication, which is governed by morphological variation related to syntactic and/or semantic factors.

To give an idea of the grammatical phenomenon, Subject-verb agreement for number can be modified according to:

i) the nature of the subject: phrasal subjects, as in (35), as opposed to non-phrasal subjects, as in (36). This is exemplified in the different implementations of agreement found with coordination (Heycock and Zamparelli, 2005; Picallo, 2002):

(35) Che sia partito tardi e che sia tornato presto è/*sono un fatto molto strano
*That he left late and came back early is/*are a strange thing*

(36) Carla e Maria sono/*è buone compagne di viaggio
*Carla and Maria are/*is good travelling companions*

ii) the nature of the predicate: distributive predicates, as in 38, as opposed to non- distributive predicates:

(37) I due ragazzi cantano e ballano
The two boys sing and dance

(38) Carla e Maria sono un clown e un saltimbanco
Carla and Maria are a clown and an acrobat

iii) the subject's position and its relationship to agreement, exemplified in the difference between pre-verbal (39) and post-verbal subject agreement (40), or in terms of structural distance as in (41) and (42) :

(39) Trois filles sont arrivées
(40) Il est arrivé trois filles
(41) The queen of England is you
(42) The queen of England may be you (from: Heycok and Kroch 1999)

The present research deals with the third point. We explore some of the properties related to structural distance and examine different intervening elements. Following the psycholinguistic research on agreement we investigated the phenomenon of attraction by comparing linear intervention inside the same phrase, as in the classic attraction test with prepositional modifiers (43), and with intervening elements such as object clitics (44), also linear interveners in subject-verb agreement.

(43) $[_{Subj} \ldots N_{head} \ldots N_{mod} \ldots]$ AgrS

Il professore-SG degli studenti-PL legge-SG/* leggono-PL

*The professor of the student reads/*read*

(44) $[_{Subj} \ldots N_{head} \ldots]$ $[_{AgrOP}$ PRO $_{clitic}]$ AgrS
Il professore-SG lePL legge-SG /*leggono-PL
*The professor them reads/*read*

3. Intervention effects in psycholinguistic literature

A productive empirical foundation for studying different agreement configurations in the sentence domain is the phenomenon of attraction. Attraction is manifested when an intervening element, situated in between two elements sharing an agreement relation, and mismatched in the relevant features, attracts agreement. This is simplified in the abstract configuration in (45).

(45) **X** ... **Z** ... **Y**
$[\ldots, \varphi_{Singular}]$ $[\ldots, \varphi_{Plural}]$ $[\ldots, \varphi_{Singular}]$

*The boat of the American **soldiers** leaves in the fog*
*The boat of the American **soldiers leave** in the fog

These effects are related to locality conditions: an intervening element with certain characteristics disrupts a local relation, in this case concordance.

Much experimental work has shown that there is a proximity concord effect determined by the closest noun in elicited production of sentences such as (46) (Bock and Miller; 1991).

(46) The king of the colonies is/**are**…

A number feature is thus assumed to play different roles at different stages (and modules) of language processing. Furthermore, there are interesting kinds of evidence that the role of singular and plural is not symmetric: a greater interference of plural local nouns on singular head nouns in sentences such as (47a) than the converse (47b) has been documented both in production errors (Bock and Miller, ibidem) and in slower reading times in comprehension (Pearlmutter et al., ibidem).

(47a)*The key to the cabinets WERE …
(47b)*The keys to the cabinet WAS …

These studies consistently show between 4% and 11 % agreement errors in attraction configurations in production. This proportion is significantly higher than the baseline (no mismatched features), with most errors, as already mentioned, found in the Singular-Plural (SP) condition.

The phenomenon of "attraction" seems then to be asymmetric and can be interpreted within the formalism that assumes that syntactic features are binary and implemented in terms of a marked value possessing a distinctive property, in this case (+ number), and an unmarked one (-number) lacking that property (Jakobson, 1957).

Attraction has been studied mainly in production and the asymmetry has been interpreted within the "marking and morphing" model (Bock and Eberhard, 1993) as arising at the morphological level, responsible for the morphemic building of the output speech, and due to interference within a "reconciliation" process responsible for the link between a marking stage, assumed to be notional in nature, and the lower level morphing stage.

A similar explanation for data on comprehension has been proposed by Pearlmutter et al. (1999), who assume that comprehension difficulties in sentences with singular head and plural local nouns arise from inadvertent head-overwriting on an on-the-fly NP number computation rather than a backtracking mechanism, leading to the supposition that number is syntactically considered only when a plural feature is encountered[1].

---

[1] The fact that asymmetry between singular and plural has always been tested in this particular environment, where structural locality and linear precedence conflict, leaves open many possible explanations for the level of processing at which the feature asymmetry originates, in particular whether the need for notional assignment of number to phrases plays a role. An interesting datum comes from a recent study on DP-Noun number violation in Italian, (Vespignani, 2006). In this study, using event related potential (ERPs), an asymmetry arises in parsing

In studies on the impact of syntactic factors on agreement errors interesting data come from intervention effects in English (Bock and Cutting, 1992). They observed that attraction is significantly lower in (48b) compared to (48a).

(48) a. [The editor of the history books] is/are…
b. [The editor] who rejected the books is/are…

This experiment suggests that there is a major processing difficulty in the regulation of relations between elements that are structurally similar and part of the same syntactic phrase, as in 48a. This evidence confirms that constituents are the relevant unit over which agreement takes place. In 48b the intervening phrase, *the books*, is part of the relative clause.

To understand all this evidence we can suppose that the processor, having to proceed under time pressure and with strong working memory constraints, wants clear indications of the nature of the elements to link in a local relation. When linear and hierarchical orders conflict, the system is prone to errors.

Much evidence attests to occasional subject modifier interference with verb agreement when there is a number mismatch with the head noun. However, number features within the VP have rarely been studied. A recent study on the structural properties of agreement shows different effects in term of different syntactic relations: linear precedence and hierarchical order (Franck et al. 2007). Franck et al. investigated attraction with a subject modifier in canonical Subject-Verb (SV) sentences (49a), compared with attraction in sentences with inversion of constituents, Verb-Subject order (VS):

(49a)$[_{Subj} \ldots N_{head} \ldots N_{mod} \ldots]$ AgrS
(49b)AgrS…$[_{Subj} \ldots N_{head} \ldots N_{mod} \ldots]$

---

agreement violations, for example, *Il cani / *I cane. In particular, a clear indicator of grammatical violation (a LAN + P600) arises in the PS condition (as in *I cane). In comparison, a less distinct P600 was found in thc SP condition. This kind of evidence concerning violations of the AGREE operation could show that a different effect is found in structures where a grammatical feature needs to be licensed, and opens up the possibility of a more detailed explanation of ERP components. In my opinion a number feature marked on nouns plays a different role from an agreement feature marked in the determiner, in line with Chomsky's distinction of interpretable features vs. uninterpretable. This kind of speculation makes precise predictions not yet tested.

In this experiment they found a significant reduced effect in the VS condition where intervention in terms of precedence is non-active. In the present study we replicate this effect with our patient.

In addition, they investigated attraction effects with two different classes of interveners: prepositional modifiers and clitic object pronouns in French.

(50a) [$_{\text{Subj}}$... N $_{\text{head}}$...N$_{\text{mod}}$...] AgrS
(50b) [$_{\text{Subj}}$...N$_{\text{head}}$...] [$_{\text{AgrOP}}$ PRO $_{\text{clitic}}$] AgrS

The main finding of this experiment is a significant number of attraction errors with clitics compared with prepositional modifiers. They explained this effect by differences in the structural relations involved. In 50b the intervening constituent, the clitic, is in a c-command relationship with the agreement head and not only in a configuration of linear precedence, as in (50a).

They also found that plural head nouns generated more errors than singular head nouns, as did plural intervening elements compared with singular ones. As we showed above, this effect is attested in other studies, suggesting that plural nouns are marked forms and they are better interveners.

In Dutch (Hartsuiker, R.J. et al. 2001) it was found that number features on preverbal objects in embedded clauses (linearly intervening between subject and verb) cause attraction effects. Effects were reported with both full NPs (51a) and with weak pronouns (51b).

(51) a. Karin says that the girl the garlands WIN
Karin zegt dat het meisje de wedstrijd wint
b. Karin says that the captain them ATTACK
Karin zegt dat de kapiteijn hen aanvalt

These pre-verbal objects were found to disrupt agreement less than subject modifiers (a PP internal to the subject phrase). Interestingly, not all pronouns show equal effects: ambiguously case-marked pronominal objects ("*ze*", 'them' for inanimate objects) induced more agreement errors than pronouns unambiguously marked for non-nominative case ("*hen*", 'them' for animate objects). The first type induces as many errors as the corresponding full NP condition.

In German, agreement errors were elicited on subject modifiers with different prepositions. It was found that accusatives induced more errors than non-ambiguous datives.

(52) *Die stellungname gegen die demonstationen*
The comment on the demonstrations

One possible explanation is that the local noun takes the accusative case depending on the preposition (importantly, the accusative case marker is not distinguishable from the nominative case marker). Case marking for dative is transparent and induces fewer errors.

Other interesting data come from Spanish. Crucially for the present investigation, manipulation of clitic object pronouns reveals no attraction effects in Spanish (Anton-Mendez, 1996). Spanish differs from other Romance languages in that it lacks participial agreement, and therefore the head for object agreement. These data show that the differences between the languages investigated may be related to grammatical selection. In other words, a non-active agreement position in a language does not induce attraction effects. This evidence will be relevant for the analysis of the present case study.

In Italian attraction effects in subject-verb agreement when the intervener is an object clitic should be more similar to the effects found in French than those in Spanish. This is because French and Italian have object agreement but Spanish doesn't (see the examples in (53)). In French, as in Italian but not Spanish, the clitic pronoun is an active element for agreement. This can be seen in past participle agreement with a preverbal object clitic.

(53a) Les pommes, je **les** ai mang**ées**
(53b) Le mele **le** ho mangiat**e**
(53c) Las manzanas **las** he comido [No Agr]
The apples, I them have eaten

Instead, object clitics intervention with the attraction paradigm revealed a kind of intermediate pattern for Italian (Garraffa and coll., 2010). More precisely, unlike in Spanish, attraction occurs when a plural object clitic intervenes between a subject and the verb. However, comparison of the two conditions shows that in Italian, unlike in French, there is a less pronounced effect with object clitics than with prepositional modifiers. To understand this intermediate pattern in Italian better, it is necessary to adduce a new element in the discussion on grammatical agreement. An explanation needs to be found for the fact that fewer attraction effects with object clitics than with prepositional modifiers where found in Italian while Franck et al. found the opposite pattern in French. We take the view that cross-linguistic differences play an important role in agreement operations. The attraction paradigm is a useful instrument for testing subtle distinctions between languages in grammatical processing.

Romance languages have rich pronominal systems, which have been extensively investigated in linguistic theory (for an overview see Cardinaletti and Starke, 1999). Pronouns divide into three different classes according to their grammatical properties: clitics, weak pronouns and strong pronouns. These categories are fairly fluid and the number of pronouns in each class differs according to language. More simply, clitics are nominal arguments closely linked with the verbal domain. In Italian, the pronominal argument moves to AgrO, the landing site for clitics, as a head, as illustrated in (54) (see Belletti, 1999 for all formal details).

(54)

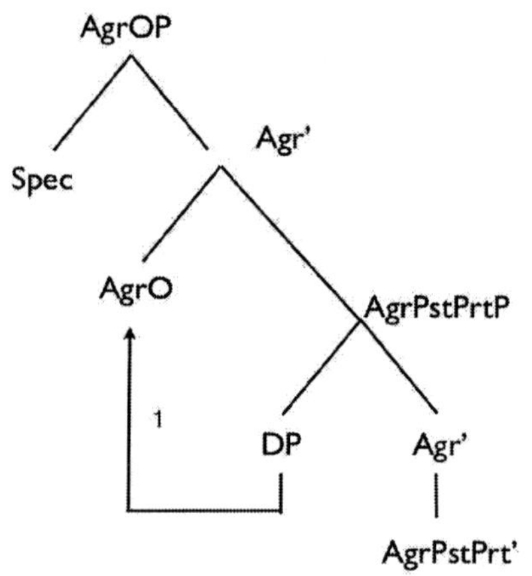

Belletti (ibidem) argues that the status of object clitics is different in French. In particular, the pronominal object DP moves to the AgrO phrase as a maximal projection and not as a simple head. This is illustrated in (55), which shows a comparison of Italian (1) and French (2) object pronouns, according to Belletti.

(55)

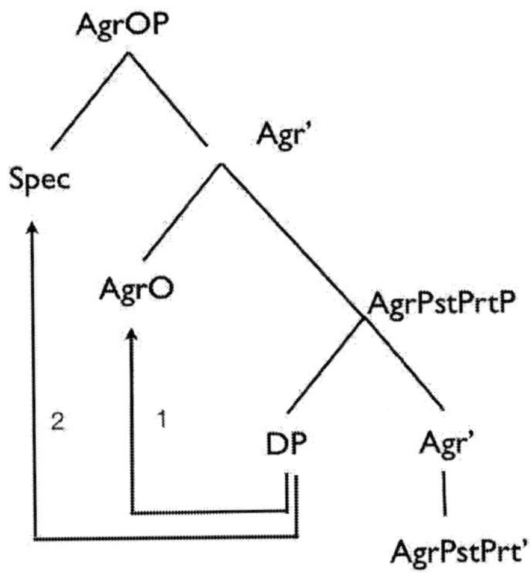

Belletti refers to cross-linguistic differences in the Romance languages in support of this analysis. For example, in non-finite constructions we find proclisis in French, whereas in Italian we find enclisis of the pronoun, a closer relationship with the verb.

(56) Les voir	proclisis in French
(57) Vederle	enclisis in Italian

Kayne (1991) makes another interesting observation regarding French, which is that in particular contexts it is possible to disrupt the continuum between an object pronoun and the verb, as in (57).

(57) Pour le bien faire
...en bien parler (Kayne, 1991)

It is possible that French object clitics, being more similar to weak pronouns, have a different internal structure and hence give rise to more attraction errors. Absence of misanalysis in Italian is limited to the few instances of weak pronouns, that is, the dative pronoun *loro* ('to them').

In Italian, clitics differs from prepositional modifiers in that they are not DPs but simply nominal heads, and hence they do not have the same structure as the agreement source, the subject DP. Clitics have a different structure to subjects and do not induce attraction in Italian.

(58)

	X ...	Z ...	Y
	[...,[-num]]XP	[...,[+num]]**X°**/XP	[...,[-num]]
	Il professore	li	legge
	The teacher	*them*	*read*

It is possible that French clitics are interpreted as DPs, and hence of the same grammatical class as subjects, and it is therefore clear why they induce attraction effects. This does not happen in Italian where the principle of Minimality clearly distinguishes object clitics from subjects, which belong to different grammatical categories.

In Italian there is no proximity between the clitic, an X°, and the subject, an XP, as illustrated in 59[2].

(59)

	X ...	Z ...	Y
	[...,[-num]]XP	[..., [+num]]X°	[...,[-num]]
	L'arbitro	li	fischia

---

[2] This analysis is also supported by a recent study (Hamman and Belletti, 2008) on early and adult French L2 learners in which placement errors (pronouns produced in DP positions) were found and were put down to misclassification of the pronouns, which had been treated as weak. These errors were produced either in isolation, as in (i), after a preposition (ii), or in canonical object position (iii).

(i) E: c'est à moi, le. — Elisa 4;2 in isolation, with stress
L: le quoi?
it's to me, him/it/the
the what?
'it's mine, that' 'which?'

(ii) alors, tu joue avec le. — Elisa 4;2 after a preposition (2 occurrences)
so, you play with him/it
'so, you are playing with it'

(iii) non, on laisse le. — Elisa 4;2 in canonical object position
no, one leaves him
'no, we leave him/it alone'

In French, as we have seen, it is possible that there is a phase during acquisition where subject and object pronouns are assigned the same structure. There is no evidence to support object clitics being weak pronouns in Italian. The explanation for the misanalysis in French acquisition and for the clear attraction effects found uniquely in French is the presence of a richer system of weak pronouns, which is not the case in Italian.

(60)

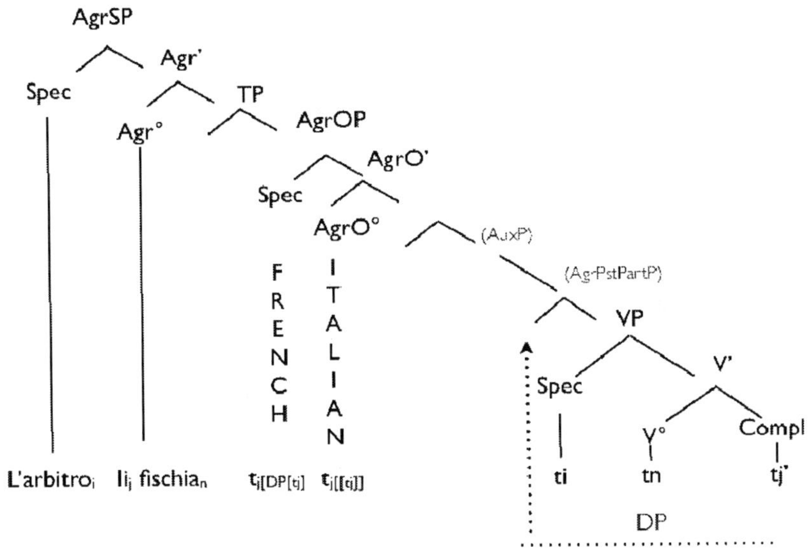

According to our initial hypothesis, subject-verb agreement should be implemented similarly in Italian and French in the condition with a clitic intervener. We now have to reconsider this hypothesis and add a new level to the analysis of this pronominal category.

As table 10 shows, object pronouns have a different status in French and in Italian, which accounts for greater attraction effects in French.

	AgrPstPrt	Weak Pronoun	Object clitic interference
ITALIAN	+	-/+	-/+
FRENCH	+	+	+
SPANISH	-	-	-

Table 10 Cross-linguistic classification for attraction effects

4. Clitics in non-fluent aphasia

Concerning clitics in aphasia, many studies have reported deficits in the production of clitic forms in aphasia. Clitic elements are impaired in agrammatic aphasia (Ferreiro, 2002; Garraffa, 2009; Nespoulous *et al.* 1988; Miceli *et al.* 1989; Reznik, et al., 1995; Stavrakaki and Kouvava

2002; Chinellato 2004; Rossi 2007; Nerantzini 2008; Tsigas 2007). Although perhaps not universally (see Chinellato (2004) on Veneto subject and object clitics), a dissociation between subject and object forms has been commonly documented (Nespoulous *et al.* ibidem; Stavrakaki and Kouvava, ibidem). In addition, some clitic types have been found to be better preserved than others, as is the case, for example, of genitive clitics in Greek, which were found to be spared more than object clitics (Stavrakaki and Kouvava, ibidem), and indirect object clitics in Italian, which were more impaired than direct object clitics (Rossi ibidem), though omission has been found to be the most common error type.

Interesting data for a definition of clitic disruption in aphasia related to syntactic computation comes from an extensive study on clitics with Italian aphasics (Rossi, 2005). The study compares Italian speakers with a group of Italian aphasic patients. In this study agrammatic patients produced significantly fewer clitics than control subjects. Different clitic contexts were also investigated: enclisis and proclisis. These contexts were tested with modals verbs. In Italian in a configuration where a non-finite verb is governed by a modal verb clitics can appear in either position, as shown in (61a) and (61b).

(61a) Maria *la* vuole suonare
Maria it want to play
(61b) Maria vuole suonar*la*
Maria want to play it

As proposed in the literature (Cardinaletti and Slonsky, 2004) clitic climbing is optional. The pronoun can occupy two different positions: an IP position connected to functional verbs and a position related to lexical verbs. Only the first position is compatible with clitic climbing. Eleonora Rossi tested this with a sentence completion task involving object clitics (accusatives and datives) in sentences where clitic climbing is mandatory.

(62a)Ieri Maria la ha mangiata, ma oggi Maria non … [la mangia]
Yesterday Maria it has eaten, but today Maria doesn't .....[it eat]
(62b)Maria non vuole mangiarla invece Gianni la vuole mangiare/vuole mangiarla
Maria not wants to-eat-it but Gianni it wants to-eat / wants to-eat-it

Interestingly, in (62b) patients preferred an enclitic configuration. They did not manifest clitic climbing. Of more relevance to our study is that in

the proclitic configuration of (62b) the most frequent error was substitution of gender and number features.
Even more relevant for the present discussion is Tsigas's extensive study on clitics in Cypriot-Greek (Tsigas, *ibidem*). Agrammatic Cypriot speakers produced fewer clitics in post-verbal position than pre-verbally. Following the base generated hypothesis (Marinis, 2000), clitics in Cypriot-Greek are generated in pre-verbal position, and the post-verbal positioning arises when the verb moves to check functional features (see Marinis, *ibidem* for a detailed description).This means that the post-verbal construction is more problematic since it is derived by movement, while clitics in Cypriot-Greek are base-generated in preverbal position. A possible solution would be to explore the idea that in Cypriot-Greek clitics in preverbal position are more similar to weak pronouns. This idea needs to be considered in further research.
Other interesting data from studies of clitics in aphasic patients comes from an investigation of comprehension of sentences with ditransitve verbs in 11 Italian agrammatic patients (Luzzatti et al., 2001). They tested comprehension of passive sentences and of different clitic configurations: direct object clitics and indirect object clitics. (ScliticVt vs. SclVDOt), as in (63a) and (63b).

(63a) Maria la cerca
Maria her seeks
(63b) Maria le da un regalo
Maria to-her gives a present

The sentences with the direct object clitic are well comprehended by the patients, performance being above chance level. Performance with cliticized indirect objects, however, is not standard and below chance level. Furthermore, there is an interesting correlation. In general, non-standard performance is found with indirect object clitics and with passives. These data could be interpreted as negative correlation of the two conditions. Furthermore, three subjects in this study (C.M., E. Be. and F.C.) manifested a positive correlation: a good performance on passives and on indirect objects clitics.

The most problematic configuration in Luzzatti et al.'s study is when a potential intervener, for a example a direct object, of the relevant relation is crossed by the cliticization of the indirect object, inducing minimality effects (the basic linear order is Subj>DirtectObj >InderctObj).

(64) X Z Y
Maria le da un regalo *t*
Maria to-her gives a present t

This speculation on intervention effects needs more refinement and in the next chapter we will introduce other data compatible with this view.

5. The task

The experiment consisted of a series of auditory grammaticality judgment tasks. M.R. had to judge the grammaticality of a battery of sentences, composed of three different sets of propositions. Half the items were grammatical and half were ungrammatical.
The first set involved agreement in SubjV and VSubj configurations, such as (65) and (66).

(65a)La nave parte/*partono
*The boat leaves/*leave*

(65b)Le navi partono/*parte
The boats leave/leaves

(66a) Parte /*partono la nave
*Leaves/*leave the boat*

(66b) Partono/*Parte le navi
*Leave/*Leaves the boats*

A total of 128 items were presented, 32 in each of the four conditions (SubjV, *SubjV, VSubj, *VSubj).

The second set consisted of a list of sentences containing intervening prepositional modifiers and either pre- or post-verbal subjects, such as in (67) and (68). Two types of effect were tested with these sentences: attraction by an intervening prepositional modifier and the predicted absence of attraction in sentences with post-verbal subjects due to non-linear intervention.

[Subj- PP -VP]
(67a)L'autista dei ministri guida/*guidano con prudenza
*The driver of the ministers drives/*drive with caution*

(67b)Gli autisti del ministro guidano/*guida con prudenza
*The drivers of the minister drive/*drives with caution*

[VP - Subj – PP]
(68a)Guida/*guidano con prudenza l'autista dei ministri
Drives/drive with caution the driver of the ministers

(68b)Guidano/*guida con prudenza gli autisti del ministro
Drive/drives with caution the drivers of the minister

This set consisted of 40 items in each of the 4 conditions (SubjPPV, *SubjPPV, VSubjPP, *VSubjPP), totaling 160 items.

The third set was composed of sentences with complement clitic interveners. In this test we investigated the intervention of an element in a local structural relation and non-linear intervention in VSubj sentences, such as in (69) and (70) respectively.

[Subj-Clitic-VP]
(69a)Il corridore li supera /*superano
*The runner them overtakes /*overtake*

(69b)I corridori lo superano/*supera
*The runners him overtake/*overtakes*

[Clitic-VP-Subj]
(70a)Li supera/*superano il corridore
*Them overtakes/*overtake the runner*

(70b) Lo superano/*supera I corridori
*him overtake/*overtakes the runners*

A total of 160 items were presented, 40 in each of the 4 conditions (SubjcliV, *SubjcliV, cliVSubj, *cliVSubj). All the verbs selected are optionally transitive in Italian (for example, *guidare* 'to drive', *superare* 'to overtake'). Only direct object complement clitics were tested; indirect objects were not included in the list. A summary of the various conditions and the number of items per condition is presented in Table 11.

Inversion	Gram	VS	PP	Clitic	Total
+	+	32	40	40	112
-	-	32	40	40	112
-	+	32	40	40	112
+	-	32	40	40	112
		128	160	160	448

Table 11 Experimental conditions and items per conditions

Inversion refers to those items with a subject in post-verbal position. Grammaticality refers to the well-formedness of the sentences. VSubj/PP/Clitic are the three variables investigated, respectively the baseline with no intervention, intervention of a prepositional modifier and intervention of a clitic. All conditions were balanced in number mismatches (half the items were Singular/Plural and half were Plural/Singular).

As filler items we selected two different sentence types. For the clitic condition we used sentences with reflexive pronouns, as in (71a). For the prepositional modifier condition we used items with either the same number feature or uninflected words, such as in (71b).

(71a)Le verdure fresche **si** vendono al mattino
The vegetables fresh ***refl.*** *sell in the morning*
(71b)Il maglione **di lana** scalda
The sweater of wool keeps-warm

The experiment with M.R. was run over ten sessions. In each session a proportional number of experimental sentence types was presented in randomized order.

A control baseline was run in order to test the two attraction conditions without agreement mismatches:

Singular-Singular [SS] and Plural-Plural [PP], as in (72) and (73).

(72a)Il cane del ragazzo morde/*mordono
*The dog of the boy bites/*bite*

(72b)I cani dei ragazzi mordono/*morde
*The dogs of the boys bite/*bites*

(73a)Le scimmie li saltano/*salta
*The monkeys them jump-over /*jumps-over*

(73b)La scimmia lo salta/*saltano
*The monkey him jumps-over/*jump-over*

M.R. showed little difficulty with the control experiment. She performed the tasks in the SS and PP conditions without a significant number of errors (2/40). This is important as it shows that a general difficulty in judging ungrammatical items can be excluded as a potential bias factor.

6. Results

In this section we report the results of the grammaticality judgment tasks separately for the three conditions: agreement in SubjV vs. VSubj structures, attraction with a prepositional modifier and attraction with an object clitic. The unimpaired control participants, matched for age and education, performed at ceiling in all conditions.

6.1 Agreement in VSubj and SubjV sentences

In the first experiment M.R. performed well with only 12/128 errors (9.3%). The task is simple to perform since it involves judging the grammaticality of three-word sentences.

	Inversion	Gram	Errors	%	Sentences
SV	-	+	0/32	0	La nave parte/Le navi partono *The boat leaves/The boats leave*
*SV	-	-	2/32	6.2	*Le navi parte/ *La nave partono **The boats leaves/*The boat leave*
VS	+	+	0/32	0	Parte la nave/Partono le navi *Leaves the boat/Leave the boats*
*VS	+	-	10/32	31.2	*Parte le navi/* Partono la nave **Leaves the boats/*Leave the boat*
	Total		12/128	9.3	

Table 12. M.R.'s performance on SV-VS grammatical judgments

The majority of errors were found with sentences featuring ungrammatical post-verbal subjects (*VSubj) (10/32; 31.2%). Performance differed significantly from chance level in this condition (z-score (1) = 2.12, p. <

.025) and also differed significantly from the grammatical VSubj condition ($\chi2(1)$= 9.6, p. < 0.05). The difference between the two ungrammatical conditions, *SubjV and *VSubj, was also significant ($\chi2(1)$ =5, p. < 0.05).

6.2 Intervention with prepositional modifiers

The second experiment tested accuracy with an intervening prepositional modifier. M.R.'s responses show attraction effects with grammatical SPPV items, 10/40 errors (25%) with performance above chance level (z-score (1) = 3.16, p. < .005).

	Inver	Gram	Errors	%	Sentences
SPPV	-	-	10/40	25	La nave dei soldati parte/ Le navi del soldato partono *The boat of the soldiers leaves/The boats of the soldier leave*
*SPPV	-	+	19/40	47.5	*Le navi del soldato parte/*La nave dei soldati partono **The boats of the soldier leaves/*The boat of the soldiers leave*
VSPP	+	+	6/40	15	Parte la nave dei soldati/Partono le navi del soldato *Leaves the boat of the soldiers/Leave the boats of the soldier*
*VSPP	+	-	27/40	67.5	*Parte le navi del soldato/*Partono la nave dei soldati **Leaves the boats of the soldier/*Leave the boat of the soldiers*
	Total		62/160	38.7	

Table 13. M.R.'s performance on SPPV–VSPP

With respect to subject-verb inversion, performance in the grammatical condition, VSubjP, was above chance level with 6/40 (15%) errors (z-score (1) = 4.42, p. < .005). There were significant differences between the two inverted conditions, VSubjPP and *VSubjPP, ($\chi2(1)$ = 20.6319,p. < 0.05). In the ungrammatical inverted condition, *VSubjP, a high error rate of 27/40 (67.5%) (z-score (1)= 2.21, p < . 025) was found, with performance below chance level.

6.3 Intervention with complement clitics

The third experiment investigated agreement in attraction configurations with a clitic intervener.

	Inver	Gram	Errors	%	Sentences
ScliV	-	+	4/40	10	Il corridore li supera /I corridori lo superano *The runner them overtakes/The runners him overtake*
*ScliV	-	-	18/40	45	*I corridori lo supera/*Il corridore li superano **The runners him overtakes/*The runner them overtake*
cliVS	+	+	4/40	10	Lo superano I corridori/Li supera il corridore *Him overtake the runners/Them overtakes the runner*
*cliVS	+	-	19/40	47.5	*Lo supera i corridori/*Li superano il corridore **Him overtakes the runners/*Them overtake the runner*
	Total		45/160	28.1	

Table 14. M.R.'s performance on S-clitic-V sequences.

Four out of 40 (10%) errors were found with the pre-verbal grammatical items, SubjcliV. Performance was above chance level (z-score (1)b =5.05,p. >.005) and differed significantly from performance in the ungrammatical condition, *SubjcliV, (χ2(1)= 10.5956, p. < 0.05).
Few errors (4/40, 10%) were also found with the grammatical inverted items, cliSubjV. Here again, performance differed significantly from the ungrammatical inverted condition, *cliVSubj X, (χ2(1) = 11.9603 p. < 0.05).

7. General discussion

In this experiment we used attraction effects in a variety of configurations to study M.R.'s perception of grammaticality with respect to agreement. This experimental stratagem was very productive, resulting in significant effects due to the non-standard condition of our subject.

M.R.'s performance clearly shows attraction effects in [S-PP]-V configurations. These effects were significantly higher than those generally obtained in the adult system. It is interesting to note that her performance on this task is at chance level (47,5%). In normal adults for Italian the occurrences of errors in attraction are around 16 %.

We can interpret these results as a consequence of minimality effects induced by the agreement feature of the intervening prepositional modifier.

(74) **X** … **Z** … **Y**

$[\ldots,\varphi_{Singular}]$ $[\ldots,\varphi_{Plural}]$ $[\ldots,\varphi_{Singular}]$

M.R. is considering both nouns as possible antecedents for the agreement relation with the verb. We can suppose that in a situation in which the processing cost is high (maintaining two agreement realizations before the verb form) the system is prone to error, and in damaged subjects performance can drop to chance level. We will develop this argument in chapter 5, presenting results from other experiments on comprehension displaying a similar pattern.

M.R. (unlike the adult French speakers tested by Frank et al., 2006) does not show any attraction with a clitic intervener. This might seem surprising at first sight since the clitic intervenes not only linearly but also hierarchically. In the study on French adults the mechanism to implement agreement seems to be influenced by local constituents: more attraction effects occur with a clitic intervener.

Crucially, no effect was found in Spanish (Antón-Méndez, 1996) where the local elements were object clitics marked with accusative case.

The absence of attraction effects with an object clitic in the Spanish case and in our Italian aphasic speaker can be accounted for.

The attraction effect is the result of an analysis of syntactic structure applied to abstract representations. We found attraction to be sensitive to categorial distinctions and to indicate subtle cross-linguistic distinctions in the pronominal systems of Romance languages. Fewer attraction effects were found with clitics than with prepositional modifiers, since there are no weak subject pronouns in Italian and clitics must be in a local configuration with the verb. According to minimality effects these elements are different enough to be distinguished from subjects.

Another interesting observation relates to the markedness of features.

In linguistic theories the number feature of a lexical item is expressed in an autonomous phrase (a NumP, or DP itself). Agreement is a morphosyntactic operation applied in a transparent system: distinct positions in the structure (functional heads) license distinct morphosyntactic features. If a position is not given a value the element cannot check the formal feature and it maintains its default value (possibly as assigned in the lexicon, where lexical items are stored in the singular form). Nodes may be underspecified, lacking dependents entirely; in this case they take the default interpretation [3]. On the other hand, if this position is marked, a number value is added to the lexical item, which becomes [+ Number]. During on-line interpretation of the agreement between two constituents we expect the parser to be sensitive to the emptiness or not of the number head: it is possible that the number agreement between two lexical constituents is directly checked by the relative number phrases only if a number marking fills both of these positions.

Plural marking on an item $X_{[+Number]}$ pre-activates agreement-sensitive processes to check the grammatical feature of a following Y constituent. On the other hand, a lexical item $X_{[-Number]}$ does not necessarily trigger any agreement checking related to the number feature. As a consequence, stronger expectations regarding the number of a following "supposed-to-agree" constituent should produce more processing difficulties if an agreement violation is detected in this last item.

[3] This difference could be parameterized cross-linguistically. In this sense English could be the case of a non-movement language, [[D] [Num] [Noun]], while in Italian the noun could move up to Num.

CHAPTER FIVE

STRUCTURAL ASYMMETRIES IN INTERROGATIVE DEPENDENCIES

In this chapter we present M.R.'s performance on production of interrogative sentences. Since Friedmann's (1997 and related works) influential proposal that deficits are related to a structural reduction of the syntactic tree, many agrammatic patients have been tested on their production of interrogatives.

These studies have made use of specific elicitation techniques and have been run cross-linguistically in order to investigate varying grammatical properties of Wh dependencies.

In general, non-Argumental (A') dependencies seem to be problematic in agrammatic speech. The present case study reported specific asymmetries, such as selective impairment in the production of Who object questions. These data could be interpreted as an indication of a selective deficit in object WH questions, in particular those with animate arguments. Furthermore, Which-questions (Discourse Related Dependencies) confirmed a grammatically based deficit, as revealed in production with a filled gap element (as in "Quale libro hai letto un libro?", lit. "Which book did you read a book?").

M.R.'s data on Wh dependencies will be discussed in terms of minimality effects induced in intervener configurations. Specifically, the extraction of an animate object operator, Who, may be blocked by an intervention effect. This is possible because the pronominal null subject functions as a possible intervener in the relevant chain.

We will also include some important comments on task-dependent effects which emerged from our study.

1. On interrogatives in aphasia

Friedmann (2000, 2002) and Friedmann and Grodzinsky (1997, 2000) propose that agrammatic speakers' tree representations are "pruned" from the TP node up, such that the landing sites for syntactic movement are missing. Consequently, sentences that require movement to the CP layer are not produced. As evidence, Friedmann (2002) reports that Hebrew and Arabic agrammatic speakers make significantly more errors when producing WH-questions (which require movement of an operator to SpecCP) than Yes/No-questions (which do not visibly manifest movement to CP in these languages). Many data were collected to investigate this divergence in the nature of interrogatives. Friedmann (2002) presents the case of an English patient with a deficit in Yes/No questions, indicating impairment possibly due to the visible markedness of the CP layer by the auxiliary *do* This result was explained in terms of tree size, the highest nodes of the syntactic tree not being accessible to agrammatic subjects. The finding that Yes/No questions were less impaired than WH-questions was replicated in Dutch (Ruigendijk et al., 2004).

On the other hand, in a group of German patients Penke and Nehauss (2003) did not find a diverging performance on WH- vs. Yes/No questions; instead, many of the patients preserved WH-interrogatives (89-100%), in particular "What-object" questions. In Italian, Chinellato (2004) investigated a group of non-fluent speakers. He found two kinds of WH operators preserved: "*Why*" and "*What*". It is interesting to note that in Italian the operator "Why" (perchè) does not activate inversion of the subject, which is obligatory with other *wh* items:

(74) Perchè Gianni ride?
Why Gianni laughs
Why does Gianni laugh?
*Dove Gianni va?
Where Gianni goes
Dove va Gianni?
Where goes Gianni
Where is Gianni going?

In Rizzi (1997) it was suggested that "Why" is a base-generated operator in the CP layer, while all the others operators reach the periphery only after movement. In a study on Iberian patients (Martinez, 2007) and in my dissertation on an Italian patient (Garraffa, 2003) the same pattern of a preserved "Why" construction was observed.

The second preserved WH dependencies in Chinellato's study are non-animate object questions: "What-object". These findings were replicated in Penke's study on German and in the present study, and are crucial for our approach to sentence production. We will address this point in greater depth in the analysis of M.R.'s data.

An interesting finding with respect to interrogatives in aphasics comes from a study on Norwegian dialects (K. Berntzen and A. Hestvik, 2003). Norwegian dialects differ from English both with respect to tree size and with respect to verb movement. The Northern and some Western dialects do not require verb movement in WH- questions when the WH- word is "light", e.g. *"Ka du sa?" "Kor du satt?"*. According to the standard analysis of Norwegian dialects for "economy of projection" principles these interrogatives only project a C', but without V-movement. The WH-word is in C°:

(75) [C' kai [IP du sa ti]]

However, if the adjunct or object is morphologically complex or phrasal the WH-phrase must move to SpecCP; thus verb movement is required and a CP is projected, as in "*Katti kom du*?" *"Ka slags Hus bor du i?":*

(76) [CP kattii [C' komv [IP du tv ti]]].

Furthermore, subject questions move WH to SpecCP but do not require verb movement, inserting instead a complementizer in C°, irrespective of WH-type, as in *"Kem som kom?"*,*"Ka slags dyr som skrek?"*. This results in a CP without V-movement:

(77) [CP Kem [C' som [IP t kom]]]

In summary, there are three categories of interrogatives: C' with no verb movement (75); CP plus verb movement (76), and CP without verb movement (77). The tree-pruning theory predicts that categories (76) and (77) should be harder to process than category (75). However, another influential theory in agrammatic aphasia (Bastianse et al., 2002) regarding deficits in verb movement predicts that (77) should be harder to process than (75) and (76). In Bastianse et al.'s experiment seven male aphasic patients were tested and it was found that their production difficulties with WH- questions could not be accounted for by differences in tree structure size. However, if the sentence requires verb movement in addition to XP-movement, the performance of the subjects becomes significantly worse.

The current findings are in agreement with Bastiaanse and Thompson's (2002) claim that agrammatics are specifically impaired with respect to verb movement.

Many studies have also been run on the comprehension of *WH*-questions. English shows subject/object asymmetries (Thompson et al., 1999) but, unfortunately, Yes/No questions were not examined in this study.

Further interesting data come from a study on French/Quebec patients (Van der Meulen, 2005).Two main findings emerge from this study: easier comprehension of interrogatives with the object in-situ than with fronted objects, and a high degree of impairment in the comprehension of *who* subject questions.

French exhibits complementizer agreement only in subject-extraction cases. This pattern is also seen in the productions of some children who produce medial *Wh* questions. In French the complementizer "*que*" changes to "*qui*" by Spec/Head agreement (for details see Rizzi 1990). This phenomenon ensures that there is a proper head governor in embedded interrogatives.

(78) Que crois-tu qui t est arrive?
What think-you that t has happened?
What do you think has happened?

The data reported in the study on French patients are important since they support the idea of a subject/object asymmetry. In Van der Meulen's approach the disturbance in agrammatic comprehension is related to featural movement.

We can conclude that A' positions share operator features with their heads. These positions are landing sites for quantifier expressions such as WH operators and topicalized elements (see Rizzi, 2002 for more details).

Syntactic constructions featuring these positions, for example relative clauses and interrogatives, seem particularly problematic for agrammatic patients. As we will see in the discussion, data from neuropsychology are also relevant to the issue.

2. The experiment

In light of the difficulties M.R has in producing full sentences in normal conversation, we adopted an elicited production technique in order to investigate her production abilities. Furthermore, with this methodology the exact target item can be reconstructed and lexical retrieval effects can be excluded, since all the words will have already been presented in the experimental context.

The technique involves the patient participating in a game aimed at eliciting the relevant syntactic structure, which is otherwise rare in spontaneous speech.

The experiment comprised 132 questions divided over three categories: *Yes/No* questions, *Who/What* questions and *Which*-x referential questions. Details of the experimental material are presented below.

132 items
Yes/No questions: 36 items, 18 with the auxiliary TO BE and 18 with TO HAVE

Who/What questions: 54 argument *Wh* items: 24 subjects, 24 objects;
24 *Wh* subjects: 12 *Who* [+animacy], 12 *What* [-animacy];
24 *Wh* objects: 12 *Who* [+animacy], 12 *What* [-animacy],

Which-x questions: 48 argument items:
24 *Wh* subjects: 12[+ animacy], 12[– animacy];
24 *Wh* objects: 12 [+ animacy], 12 [-animacy].

All the items were constructed to test specific grammatical properties and the experimental lists were controlled for possible biases: plausibility of the event, variation in auxiliary verb forms (*essere* has a richer morphology then *avere*), and number of verbal arguments.

We wanted to test all question types in order to exclude a possible deficit related to pragmatic factors. Since *Yes/No* questions do not involve *WH*-elements, a deficit of these closed class grammatical items would result in a good performance on *Yes/No* questions but impairment in retrieval of interrogative elements.

Constituent interrogatives involve two different types of WH-element: bare WH-elements (*Who*, *What*, *Where*, *How*, *Why*, *When*) and WH-elements of the *Which*-X type. In the generative linguistic literature the latter are referred to as Discourse Linked. These grammatical operators are licit in sentences where the range of the variable is a set introduced in the discourse. In addition to their discourse properties, D-linked elements share a set of syntactic properties. For example, D-linked *WH*-questions seem to constitute an exception to so-called Superiority:

(79)Which fruit did which person eats —?
(80)*What did who eat?

In (79) a D-linked *WH*-element can be extracted across another *WH* element of the same type. This is not possible for bare interrogative elements, as in (80).

Rizzi (1990) proposed that a *WH*-phrase with a referential argumental theta role can undergo long extraction out of a weak island, without cyclic movement, associating with its variables via binding. Cinque (1990) refined Rizzi's proposal, arguing that only *Which*-N *WH* phrases are coreferential.

Interesting experimental data comes from a study on question production in child language acquisition (Thornton, 1995). In this extensive research on 4-year-old children's interrogatives optional non-adult variations of WHICH questions were found. These grammatical options are expressed by the presence of a *medial wh*. The same option seems available for children's referential matrix questions, as in (81).

(81) Which mouse do you think [$_{CP}$who[$_{IP}$the cat chased t]]
(Example from Thornton, 1995)

Thornton argues that overt movement to a RefP phrase, covert in the adult system, is a possible option for the child's grammatical system. In adult grammar the movement takes place at LF. The logic of this argument is that children make overt certain distinctions that remain unexpressed in the adult systems.

Standard Italian displays a flexible word order in several constructions and a sentence like "*Chi ha visto Maria?*" (lit. Who has seen Maria?) is potentially ambiguous between a subject or an object question reading. To avoid this ambiguity the experiment was designed to force the overt presence of the second person object clitic *ti* , as in *Chi ti ha baciato?,* (lit. Who you has kissed? *Who kissed you?)*, involving the patient directly in an interview situation with the investigator. This was necessary to give the experimenter the certainty that the patient had activated the correct representation-interpretation. The clitic in fact is an important cue in disambiguating a subject from an object interpretation.

Animacy features of the WH-operators were balanced. In Italian, as in English, animacy is grammaticalized in interrogative elements. The difference between the two WH-elements *Who* and *What* is the presence/absence of the property of animacy in relation to their quantification of an argument. Basically, the WH-element *Who* is grammatically marked with a [+ animate] feature and *What* with a [-animate] feature. The reason for testing the patient's abilities with [±animate] *WH* items will be made clearer in the discussion.

2.1 Procedure

All the items were arranged into 11 different lists and each list contained all question types in randomized order, with a correction that excluded more than three of the same type in succession. The subject's task was to produce the target sentence after presentation of the relevant context.

To test competence on *WH*-dependencies we used a task developed in L1 acquisition studies (Thornton, ibidem). The context for eliciting the sentences involves a syntactic structure called *sluicing*. Sluicing is a deletion process at the level of phonetic form, resulting in a type of ellipsis (Ross, 1969). An example of this linguistic phenomenon is presented in (82):

(82) Maria visited somebody but she didn't say who <she visited>

These contexts have proved successful in testing WH-dependencies in L1 acquisition. We have adapted them for our experiment.

In the experiment developed for children the investigator tells the child a story: this is the context for elicitation. At the end of the story the investigator invites the child to ask a puppet a missing detail of the story:

(83) Investigator: "In that story, there was **something** the spaceman didn't like. Ask the snail **what_**"
Target:
What did the spaceman not like?

In the experiment created for our patient we used *sluicing* contexts, similar to those used by Thornton in L1 acquisition.Contexts and target answers are presented in (84):

(84a) WHAT-OBJECT
Investigator: Ho mangiato qualcosa di speciale. Tu vuoi sapere **cosa**.Quindi mi chiedi . . .
I ate something special. You want to know ***what****. So you ask me . . .*
Target: Cosa hai mangiato?
What did you eat?

(84b) WHO-OBJECT
Investigator: Ho incontrato qualcuno dopo il cinema. Tu vuoi sapere **chi**. Quindi mi chiedi . . .
I met someone after the cinema. You want to know ***who***. *So you ask me . . .*
Target: Chi hai incontrato?
Who did you meet?

(85a) WHAT-SUBJECT
Investigator: Qualcosa mi ha sporcata. Tu vuoi sapere **cosa**. Quindi mi chiedi . . .
Something soiled me (my clothes). You want to know ***what***. *So you ask me . . .*
Target: Che cosa ti ha sporcata?
What has soiled you?

(85b) WHO-SUBJECT
Investigator: Qualcuno mi ha salutato per la strada. Tu vuoi sapere **chi**. Quindi mi chiedi
Someone greeted me in the street. You want to know ***who***. *So you ask me . . .*
Target: Chi ti ha salutato per la strada?
Who has greeted you in the street?

The subject had to ask the question, substituting the indefinite in the first sentence with the relevant *WH* element and moving the latter to the interrogative position in the CP layer[1].

The experiment was also carried out with one control subject, paired with our aphasic subject in age, education and mother tongue (standard Italian). The procedure was the same for both subjects. The control subject did not show any deviation from the target items, confirming the validity of the technique.

The experimental sessions were fully recorded, including training sessions and conversation during pauses. The investigator read the contexts. The session did not have a time limit and the subject could ask for repetitions or could interrupt. Every session was preceded by a training session. The procedure was the same for all item types.

[1] See Garraffa (2004) for a discussion of the relevant experimental context and comparison with other techniques to elicit interrogatives.

As part of the experiment we also presented a set of real objects or pictures of people, which was necessary to create the appropriate context for D-linked elements. For example to elicit a *which*-object question as in *Which book did Maria read?* we presented the subject with a set of different books. This lends plausibility to a Discourse-linked interrogative.

3. Results

In this paragraph we present the results of the experiment. M.R.'s performance in question elicitation is summarized in Table 15.

Production	N	Correct	%
Wh- question	48	28	58.3
Yes/ No question	36	20	56
Referential- Wh question	48	31	64.5
TOT	132	79	59.8

Table 15 M.R.'s results on question elicitation

At fist sight there seems to be no particular preference for any type of interrogative, all being clearly impaired. A more in depth analysis, however, reveals interesting asymmetries. In the following sections we present the results for each question type (*Yes/No, Who/What* subject and object and *Which* subject/object) separately. As reported in Table 19 M.R. obtained low scores in all her interrogatives (56-64% correct), with little variation between the three types - *Yes/No*, *WH* and *Which-x*. This observation conflicts with data reported in the literature that show a better performance with *Yes/No* questions (Friedmann 2002; Ruigendijk et al. 2004, among others).

3.1 Yes/No Questions

We found errors in the production of *Yes/No* questions, although these were limited to auxiliary omission. The absence of functional elements, also attested in declarative sentences, does not support the idea that these errors are structure dependent. Furthermore, auxiliary omission in M.R.'s questions seems sensitive to the type of auxiliary. "*essere*" (to be) is more prone to omission than "*avere*" (to have).

Yes/No	N	Correct	%	Aux Omission
To be	18	6	33.3	12
To have	18	14	77.7	4

Table 16. Auxiliary omission in Yes/No questions

With "*Avere*" (to have) interrogatives (14/18 target response) there is a significant above chance performance ($\chi(1) = 4.5$ $p < 0.05$). "*Essere*" (to be) performance is not statistically significant 6/18 (χ (1) =1.38 $p < 0.2$).

3.2 Wh Questions: Subject vs. Object

Clear asymmetries, relating to the grammatical arguments, were found in M.R.'s performance. Subject questions show fewer errors than object questions. These observations concern bare WH questions and referential questions. The two tables below summarized the relevant results.

WH – Questions	N	Correct	%
Who- subject	12	9	75
Who– object	12	0	0
What– subject	12	10	83.3
What- object	12	9	75
TOTAL	**48**	**28**	**58.3**

Table 17. M.R.'s interrogatives with *Wh* operators

REFERENTIAL questions	N	Correct	%
Subject	24	19	79
Object	24	13	54.1
Tot	**48**	**31**	**64.5**

Table 18. M.R.'s interrogative with *Which* operators

M.R. showed close-to-normal performance with subject *WH*s (75/ 83% correct). Her performance is at its worst with *Who*-object questions (no correct productions). There is considerable variation in M.R.'s performance on object questions: all of the questions with *Who* showed errors (0% correct), yet the same constructions with *What* are produced correctly in 75% of cases. The feature ±animate (all that differentiates the two *Wh* types) seems to have a strong influence on M.R.'s performance.

M.R.'s performance on questions is clearly far from standard.

Her interrogative production has many interesting aspects which call for careful explanation and which also open up avenues of future research building on the present study. The emergence of asymmetries between the different types of interrogatives, as well as the different types of error found in MR's production make a cross-modal analysis worthwhile.

Correct	Who	What	%
Subject	9/12	10/12	79.1
Object	0/12	9/12	37.5
%	37.5	79.1	

Table 19. M.R.'s scores on Who/What questions

The relevant data obtained from the production task show a selective preference for subject constituent questions and non-standard performance on object questions with a [+animate] *Wh* operator. Object Who and object What question are statistically significant $\chi^2(1) = 11.3778$, $p < 0.05$). A qualitative analysis of results is necessary to better understand M.R. errors.

With Who-subject questions she produced 3/12 that were deviant from target items.

Who subject question error types:

2 clitic omission: Chi (ti) ha accompagnato?; Chi (ti) ha salutato?

1 fragment: Chi è? *Who is?*

With *Who* object questions the patient shows 0/12 target responses, a below chance performance ($\chi^2(1) = 10.08$, $p> 0.05$). The main error type is agreement substitution (with or without clitic insertions) that generates a grammatical subject question. This is an indication of a clear preference for *who* subject interpretation[2].

Who object errors types:

9 agreement substitution: Chi ha invitato? instead of Chi hai invitato? ; in 4 productions with a clitic insertion, as in Chi ti ha salutato? instead of Chi hai salutato?

2 fragment: as Chi? Chi ha?

1 Yes/No question: hai spinto qualcuno?

[2] It is important to keep in mind that all types of items are equally presented in every session; this is why it would hardly be possible to interpret these data as an effect of simple repetition of the same question type, e.g. always a subject one.

What subject questions were significantly above chance (($\chi^2(1)= 4.08$, $p > 0.05$).

What subject error types:
1 clitic omission: Cosa ha macchiato? instead of Cosa ti ha macchiato?
1 fragment: Cosa?

What object error types:
1 agreement substitution: Che cosa ha macchiato? Instead of Che cosa hai macchiato?
1 fragment:Che cosa è? instead of che cosa studi?
1 substitution with a Yes/No question: hai mangiato? instead of Che cosa hai mangiato?

It is relevant to underline for the present analysis that M.R. does not show a deficit in checking agreement in *what* questions, 1/12 substitution (in contrast with 9/12 substitutions presented in *who* object questions). This is an important contrast to strengthen the idea that the subject position does not count as intervener in *what* questions.

In production of Subject Which-x question we have 18 out of 24 target responses, a significant above chance performance ($\chi^2(1)=5.0417$, $p < 0.05$)

Which-x subject error typologies:
5 agreement substitution: Quale amica hai truccato? Instead of Quale amica ti ha truccata?

With Object Which-x performance we have 13 out of 24 target responses, a performance not significantly different from chance level ($\chi^2(1)= 0.0417$, $p = 0.8383$).

Which-x object error typologies:
6 filled gap, as in Quale piatto hai rotto un piatto? Which plate did you brake a plate?
5 agreement substitution: Quale bambina ha spaventato? Instead of Quale bambina hai spaventato?

4. Discussion

The correct representation of an interrogative sentence requires activation of the relevant WH feature, which in turn forces the element it is associated with to appear in its dedicated position in the left periphery. The existence of a split between lower (accessible) projections in the tree and these left peripheral (inaccessible) positions in the syntactic representation of agrammatic speakers is at the root of the influential Tree Pruning Hypothesis (Friedmann 1998, 2002).

This theory can account for some aspects of M.R.'s deficit, but certain formal features (e.g. those related to the syntax-discourse interface or to operators) are more difficult to explain in terms of a non-active syntactic tree.

A more suitable characterization of M.R.'s interrogatives emerges from a recent study on agrammatic comprehension (Grillo, 2005; Garraffa and Grillo, 2008; and chapter 6 of the present monograph).

In this approach a deficit in high-level positions of the tree structure, e.g. the CP layer, is a natural consequence of non-standard activation and representation of operator features. The possibility that effects similar to those found in comprehension could also show up in other linguistic modalities is a natural one, even taking into account plausible distinctions between production and comprehension[3].

The results presented here offer preliminary support for this claim: a substantial asymmetry arises between subject and object WH question production, objects showing more errors than subjects. When chain construction requires that an NP - a potential intervener - be crossed the patient's performance deteriorates significantly.

Sensitivity to subtle, lower level grammatical distinctions seems to play a crucial role in helping the patient construct the correct representation. In our experiment it is the mismatch in animacy between the moved object and the intervening subject, when present, which seems to be responsible for a significant increase in correct responses. We interpret this as indication of the adaptation of a grammatical principle (the condition on locality) to an exceptional situation.

4.1 Who questions

M.R.'s performance on *who* questions shows a clear asymmetry in the production of subject and object questions: the latter are much more problematic for the patient (to an extreme degree: all productions were incorrect); performance on the former is considerably better (75% correct), as reported in table 7. This asymmetry is not new in the literature on

[3] In chapter 6 we will discuss in detail Grillo's hypothesis on agrammatic comprehension.

agrammatism; see e.g. Neuhaus and Penke (2003) for similar results in a study on five German Broca's patients.

It is important to note that the *Who* object questions were not ambiguous in this task. The experiment was designed in such a way as to force the overt presence of the second person object clitic *ti* 'you' (*Chi ti ha baciato?,* lit. *Whom you have kissed?*); this was necessary in order to assure the experimenter that the patient had activated the correct representation-interpretation. The clitic, in fact, is an important cue in disambiguating between a subject and an object interpretation. This is because standard Italian has flexible word order in many constructions. For example, a sentence such as *Chi ha visto Maria?* (lit. *Who has seen Maria?*) is potentially ambiguous between a subject and an object question interpretation. Of more importance for the present analysis, M.R. does not have difficulties in producing the clitic to obtain the right subject interpretation. In *who* subject questions 9/12 of the target responses are correct.

On the other hand, with *Who* object questions the patient shows a quite systematic theta role inversion. This appears clearer when we look at the types of errors: 4 agreement substitutions, 5 agreement substitutions + clitic insertion, 2 fragments, and only 1 substitution with a Yes/No question. Agreement substitutions (with or without clitic insertions) generate a grammatical subject question, which again shows a clear preference for *who* subject interpretations[4].

A possible explanation for these data is that in a subject *who* question a problem with the representation of the operator feature should not lead to a production problem: even if this problem results in a change in the class to which the moved element belongs, the absence of any potential intervener (NP) between it and its extraction position cannot give rise to any minimality effect. In these schemas, underspecification in M.R.'s syntactic representation of a subject *who* question is compared with a normal representation.

Normal Representation

(86) a. $_{CP}$[N, +an,φs, nom, θ1,+ Wh] $_{VP}$[N, + an φs, nom, θ1,+Wh]
Chi < *Chi* > ti ha baciato ?
Who *<Who>* *you has kissed?*

[4] It is important to keep in mind that all types of items were presented in a random distribution in every session, which is why these data cannot be interpreted as an effect of repetition of a given question type, e.g. always a subject one.

Agrammatic Representation

b. $_{CP}$[N, +animate] $_{VP}$[N, + animate]
Chi < *Chi* > ti ha baciato?
Who <*Who*> *have kissed?*

The situation clearly changes when the patient is asked to produce an object question: in this case the absence of the operator feature, and the change of class (from Operator to Argument) of the set of features associated with the syntactic element to be moved, makes the intervention of the subject NP critical for minimality[5]. With object but not with subject *wh*-movement enduring activation of the probe is necessary to ensure attraction of the right goal over the intervening NP. In other words, only in this case is it necessary to keep the relevant features active and to keep the differences between the syntactic elements visible. Crucially for our discussion, the possibility of a breakdown is revealed dramatically in the asymmetry between subject and object questions: with **0%** of production of *who* object questions being correct.

Normal Representation

(87)

a.$_{CP}$[N,+an,φs,acc,θ2,+Wh] $_{IP}$[N,+an,φs,nom,θ1] $_{VP}$[N,+an,φs, acc,θ2,+Wh]
Chi *pro* hai baciato <*Chi* > ?
Who *have[2°sing] kissed* *< Who >?*

Agrammatic Representation

b. $_{?}$[+ Animate] $_{IP}$[+ Animate] $_{VP}$[+ Animate]
Chi *pro* hai baciato *< Chi > ?*
Who *have[2°sing] kissed* *< Who >?*

4.2 What questions

M.R.'s overall performance with *what* questions is rather good for both subject and object questions. In this case there is clearly no asymmetry between subject and object movement within the same construction; however, the difference between these results and those with *who*

[5] It is important to stress that these facts shed light on the nature of the relation between the lexicon (and its semantic interpretation) and the syntax of natural languages: the agrammatic patient knows what task she is asked to perform, she is also given the right lexical item by the experimenter (*who* in this case); nevertheless this is not enough for her to construct a correct syntactic representation.

questions cannot be ignored. *Who* object questions are in fact not produced at all: 0% vs. 75% of *what* object questions correct. The three errors in *what* questions are: one substitution with a Yes/No question, one fragment and one agreement substitution. It is relevant to underline for the present analysis that M.R. does not show a deficit in checking agreement in *what* questions, 1/12 substitution (in contrast with 9/12 substitutions presented in *who* object questions). This is important as it strengthens the idea that the subject position does not count as an intervener in *what* questions.

The good performance on *what* questions is striking and at first sight is problematic for the analysis proposed so far, which predicts that M.R. should fail in the task of producing these structures as she does with *who* questions. In other words, we would expect her to perform significantly better with subject than object *what* questions.

Despite the fact that we are working with agrammatic data, we are nevertheless using a 'standard version' of RM, i.e. one that has been elaborated on data from unimpaired adult speakers' grammars. We assume that in normal conditions and for an unimpaired grammar certain distinctions between syntactic elements, even grammaticalized ones, are not visible or are marginal to the instantiation of grammatical operations and boundaries (in the present case to the locality principle) because of the presence of other more 'prominent' ones.

The presence of a feature that defines a morphosyntactic feature set as belonging to the Operator class, and the existence of other differences between this element and another intervening in its 'path' and belonging to the Argumental class (e.g. differences in number and person features) are most probably disregarded by the system, in that their difference or similarity is not going to change the application of the relevant principles in any way. This state of affairs could plausibly differ in an impaired system. In this case it is possible that in order to adapt to the new situation subtler and previously ignored differences between moved NPs and other interveners in their paths could help establish the relevant dependencies.

Thus, in the case at hand we propose that the availability of a mismatch in the grammaticalized [±animate] feature can provide the system with the relevant distinctions. In the case of *what object* questions, the moved object [-animate] differs in animacy from the intervening subject [+animate]. This mismatch is irrelevant in unimpaired grammar where normal activation of the *wh*-feature allows the system to disregard these lower level distinctions. However, the same distinctions could be crucial in helping an impaired system to construct the correct syntactic representation.

Normal Representation

(88)

a. $_{CP}$[N,-An,φs,acc,θ2,+Wh] $_{IP}$[N,+An,φs,nom,θ1] $_{VP}$[N,An,φs,acc,θ2,+Wh]

Che cosa *pro* hai mangiato < *Che cosa* >?

What have eaten < *What* > ?

Agrammatic Representation

b. $_{?}$[N, -Animate] $_{IP}$[N,+Animate] $_{VP}$[N, -Animate]

Che cosa *pro* hai mangiato < *Che cosa* > ?

What have eaten < *What* > ?

If in the case of *what* questions the mismatch in animacy between the *what* object and the subject NP seems to be enough to help construct the relevant chain, the situation is quite different with *who* questions: *who* crucially shares the feature [+animate] with the intervening subject, and in this case nothing helps distinguish the two elements and the derivation crashes (see above).

4.3 Which-x questions

M.R.'s performance on *which-x* questions shows the same subject/object asymmetry found with bare *WH* phrases; the data are reported in Table 18.

Avrutin and Hickok (1995) found a similar pattern in an experiment on comprehension (with the important difference that they found above chance performance with both subject and object *who* questions).

The correct interpretation of interrogatives with Discourse-linked elements depends on the interface with extra-syntactic knowledge, which plays a crucial role in fixing the reference of the predication. In Avrutin's hypothesis processing factors are the source of the contrast between D-linked and non-D-linked dependencies. Previous accounts have claimed a difference in processing complexity between subject and object extraction (Frazier and Friederici, 1991): object extraction is more difficult to process due to the greater length of the chain. Instead, Avrutin assumes that processing overload blocks normal interpretation in both subject and object D-linked dependencies. He claims that interpretation is then handed over to a default strategy almost identical to the one posited in Grodzinsky's TDH.

We will address this point in greater detail in chapter 6 presenting data on comprehension in a framework that assumes the processing system to have an intrinsically grammatical nature.

In the present investigation an interesting error type arises from Which-x object questions. M.R. produced 6/24 (25%) filled gap constructions as in (89).

(89) *Quale piatto hai rotto un piatto?*
Which plate have [2°sing] broken a plate?

This kind of structural error is also reported in a study on Hebrew and Arabic (Friedmann, 2002): filled gap (5% in elicitation, 2% in repetition) and doubling of the WH element (5% in elicitation).

These utterances may be considered the manifestation of a structural problem in the extraction from object position. There is much of interest to speculate on regarding the nature of these utterances.

What is the nature of the critical features permitting A' dependencies?

M.R.'s non-standard interrogatives do not contain an exact copy of the interrogative phrase, as in the hypothetical utterance in 90.

(90) Quale piatto hai rotto < *quale piatto* > ?
Which plate have [2°sing] broken < which plate > ?

The utterances produced by M.R. seem to lack application of the pied-piping of the argument, where the underspecification of a particular formal feature does not permit the movement operation to be completed.

Following an argument developed in Rizzi (2000) we can assume that the special position allowing extraction from weak islands is restricted to the category DP at LF. Furthermore, Cresti (1995) argues that D-linking - while possibly favoring extraction in some contexts - is not the crucial operation. Crucial in permitting long A' dependencies is the fact that the A' trace is interpreted as an individual variable. Rizzi has rephrased reconstruction in the following terms:

> "Reconstruction is enforced by a weaker principle (a principle conceptually similar to the Avoid Pronoun Principle and other such principles of structural economy) requiring minimal Pied-Piping on LF representations". (Rizzi, 2000)

Another interesting analysis is presented in Watanabe (2006). Based on a derivational framework and on economy conditions, such as the Inclusiveness condition, he proposes that there is a formal pied-piper feature.

(91) The Inclusiveness Condition = no new features are introduced during the derivation (Chomsky, 2000,113)

Watanabe's interpretation of this condition is that the pied-piper feature should be assigned during numeration. At this point, the computational system cannot foresee which category to copy for pied-piping. The selection of this category must therefore be made when the computational system builds the structure that contains the goal for Agree as well as the pied-piper feature. If the pied-piper feature is placed in a wrong position (or is not placed at all) the computation cannot proceed any further (Watanabe, 2006).

These interrogatives could be seen as an effect of Minimal pied-piping on the LF representation where formal features related to the target position are underspecified.

Where does the distinction between the Which-x operator and Who/What come from?

In our system all of these data on question production could be interpreted as a grammatical reduction of certain formal features implemented in the syntactic tree. The empirical effect could be a reduced structure, *truncated* in Rizzi's sense.

(92)

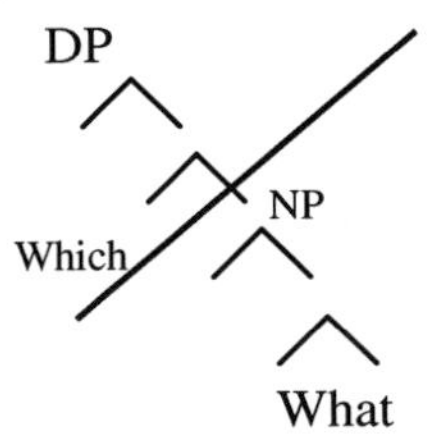

An interesting piece of linguistic evidence to support the present positional distinction comes from a study on semantic properties of the Definiteness restricition (Heim, 1987). In her investigation on *wh*-traces and definite variables Heim presents data related to the "definiteness" of the moved *wh*-phrase, (example in (93) from Heim, ibidem P. 27).

(93) a. ??Which one of the two men was there in the room/*drunk?
b. ??Which actors were there in the room/*laughing?
c. ?Who was there in the room when you got home?
d. What is there in Austin?

In essence, her argument is based on empirical observation that What-questions are not restricted to specific readings, as in dialogues like *What do you need? – A hammer.* She argues that what-questions could be analyzed as involving narrow scope similar to "something of kind x", a transparent indefinite, despite the definiteness of this kind of variable. Who has a possible intermediate state: it can mean "Which person(s)" or the interrogative counterpart of "such a person(s)", this latter option being marginally acceptable. For the aim of the present study it is relevant to underline the possible grammatical nature of this distinctions. I invite the reader to read Heim's article for in depth analysis the phenomena.

5. Summary and comments

The main argument presented in this chapter is that definition of the grammatical deficit in syntactic terms involves the notion of the chain and of minimality effects proper to the grammatical domain. In general, the definition of movement as a filler-gap relation seems inadequate and a more specific approach to chain formation is necessary to explain M.R.'s performance.

Many recent theoretical approaches highlight the necessity of addressing the fundamental duality of semantics: distinguishing argument structure from discourse-related and scopal phenomena. In this sense, the basic elements of language are chains, inasmuch as grammatical objects are able to distinguish syntactic dependencies.

In this study it was shown that movement out of an object position does not always yield a production deficit and a more finely-tuned analysis in terms of the specification of features in the syntactic tree seems to be necessary.

A comment is in order related to feature geometry and in general to the relation between formal features and lexical ones.

As has been shown here, in much of the data on aphasia formal features, and partly in parallel some aspects of the functional lexicon, are more impaired than lexical features related to content properties. This approach deals with a more general heuristic concerning the specification of information. An interesting comment related to this aspect is present in Grillo's thesis:

> "For economy reason we tend to specify more general features rather than more specific ones. This seems to be quite a natural fact regarding all other mental skills and there seems to me to exist no special reasons for language to be an exception in this sense" (Grillo, 2004 p.12)

With neurolinguistic research we have access to evidence not attested in a normal cognitive system, and what is clear in this kind of effect is that the language faculty is built on a rich set of data and simple mechanisms to decode or encode information. This could be the essence of the creativity of language.

CHAPTER SIX

CANONICITY AS A GRAMMATICAL PHENOMENON

In this chapter we present an investigation on comprehension of relative clauses. Relative clauses have been extensively investigated in the literature on agrammatic aphasia, with much discussion focused on canonical vs. non-canonical order.

The relevant variables investigated in the experiments run are word order and agreement mismatch between subject and object, allowing non-ambiguous interpretation.

In English, subject- and object-relative clauses (RCs) are disambiguated by word order: subject-RCs display the canonical SVO order, while object-RCs display a non-canonical OSV order. In Italian the sentence "Il ragazzo che ha salutato il maestro" (lit. The boy that has greeted the teacher) is potentially ambiguous. "Il maestro" could be the object of the relative clause or its post-verbal subject.

An agreement feature on the verb can disambiguate such sentences: in "I ragazzi che hanno salutato il maestro" (lit. The boys that have greeted the teacher), "il maestro" can only be the object of the relative clause, while in "I ragazzi che ha salutato il maestro" (The boys that has greeted the teacher), "il maestro" is the post-verbal subject of the relative clause. Note that with respect to the latter reading the subject of the relative clause may also appear pre-verbally: "I ragazzi che il maestro ha salutato" (lit. The boys that the teacher has greeted).

We investigated whether M.R.'s comprehension of object relatives would be less problematic when the arguments of a transitive verb, the subject and the object, differed in number features.

Furthermore, we investigated mismatches in agreement and position as possible aids to interpreting non-canonical structures in a system typically impaired with respect to the comprehension of object relative clauses.

A clear impairment occurs with non-canonical configurations. More interestingly, agreement mismatches seem to be important in helping M.R. to assign the correct thematic roles. A non-standard word order NP-NP-V and an Agreement mismatch force the grammatical system to build a syntactic chain to reach the correct interpretation. This configuration is impaired in M.R. and she does not make the correct thematic role assignments.

We will explain the pattern obtained as an effect of a reduced grammatical parsing processing.

1. On comprehension: chain specification in grammatical impairment

The existence of a discrepancy in the comprehension of semantically reversible sentences with canonical and non-canonical word order is a well-established fact since Caramazza and Zurif's seminal work (1976). The standard kind of evidence reported in many studies is summarized in Table 20.

Construction	Sentence	Performance
Active	The girl kissed the boy	**Above chance**
Subject relative	The girl who kissed the boy was tall	**Above chance**
Subject relative	Show me the girl who kissed the boy	**Above chance**
Subject cleft	It is the girl who kissed the boy	**Above chance**
Passive	The boy was inspired by the girl	**Above chance**
Passive	The boy was kissed by the girl	**Chance**
Object relative	The boy who the girl kissed is tall	**Chance**
Object relative	Show me the boy who the girl kissed	**Chance**
Object cleft	It is the boy who the girl kissed	**Chance**
Passive	The woman was unmasked by the man	**Chance**

Table 20. Sentence patterns in cross-linguistic studies on agrammatic comprehension

Divergences in the comprehension pattern have been extensively attested cross-linguistically (see, for example, Grodzinsky (2000) and the extensive commentary on the article). The empirical paradigm adopted in many studies is a picture selection task. Subjects are asked to pick out the appropriate character in a scene illustrating a sentence that is presented simultaneously. Non-standard comprehension of passive sentences, object

relative clauses and object clefts emerges, these constructions being significantly more impaired than active declaratives, subject relatives and subject clefts.

Many data supporting this pattern of impairment have been collected in agrammatic aphasia. In our view, characterization of this deficit in terms of structures, e.g. passive vs. active, is not the correct approach (see chapter 1 of the present monograph). A more in depth discussion on the source of the non-standard aphasic pattern and a clear theory on the formal aspects of the linguistic structures tested is a necessary complement to these cross-modal studies.

To understand better the present debate on agrammatic comprehension and the approach adopted in this study, we present a review of some of the relevant literature.

Different theories have been proposed to explain the empirical evidence that is often described in terms of canonical vs. non-canonical order (see Avrutin 2001 for a review)[1]. Simplifying considerably, it is possible to divide the analyses in two major classes: those describing the deficit as a loss of (part of) grammatical knowledge (Grodzinsky 1990, 1995, 2000; Friedmann 1998, 2002), and those considering it as the result of a processing deficit compromising the ability to apply such knowledge (Kolk, 1998; Haarmann and Kolk, 1992; Caplan and Hildebrandt, 1988; Just and Carpenter, 1992). These were the main proposals in the debates of the '80s and '90s and many cross-linguistic data were collected supporting one view or the other. More recently, attempts have been made to reconcile data emerging from grammatical deficits in sentence processing and to unify representational theories on linguistic competence (see the discussion in the present chapter).

A convergence of the approaches is desirable since every representational theory must at some point reflect the neuropsychological evidence, and every processing-based account must have some basis in formal linguistic terms.

For example, a recent study on the comprehension of questions in French aphasic speakers (Van der Meulen, 2004) shows that while subject interrogatives are impaired, WH questions with an in-situ object operator are comprehended correctly. The data are accounted for with a non structure-dependent explanation, but before drawing further conclusion other aspects of the language, such as the possibility of leaving the WH element in-situ, need to be looked at.

[1] Canonical order refers to Agent-first sentences. Non–canonical order is where Theme or a non-Agent thematic role is in first position.

On the other hand, Caplan (see Caplan et al.1996) has shown that when such results are combined with those of other studies, the picture that emerges is one in which the system manifests features characteristic of both distributed and localized processing.

In a recent paper, Edgar Zurif (Zurif, 2001) proposed that the discrepancy in comprehension (canonical vs. non-canonical order) has certain consequences for real-time processing. His argument is based on evidence showing slow syntactic processing in Broca's patients (see, for example, Zurif et al.1993). With a slower-than-normal activation, aphasics fail to form syntactic dependencies. Indeed, when the input rate is decreased (Swinney et al.'s (1991) experiment was run at a rate of four syllables per second compared to the normal rate of six syllables per second) Broca's patients manage to reactivate the displaced constituent in the gap-position after the verb.

Zurif has put forward a cross-disciplinary generalization, having observed a parallel between recent data from ERP studies and from neuropsychological data.

His argument is based on preliminary evidence indicating that when the input is slowed down the early left anterior negativity, ELAN, disappears. This electrophysiological signature is commonly interpreted as representing an early stage of syntactic processing, and occurs with structural violations. In models such as the one elaborated by Angela Friederici (see Friederici, 2002 for an overview) it corresponds to a first linguistic analysis of a sentence.

This syntax-first model postulates at least three temporally and spatially distinct phases of language comprehension. An early structural process subserved by the anterior part of the left hemisphere for categorical violations (the ELAN); a second post-syntactic phase where lexical-semantic and argument structure are processed, the electrophysiological correlate being distributed over the left and the right temporo-parietal areas and sometimes represented by two distinct and qualitatively different components, a syntactic LAN and a semantic N400, (but see Bornkessel and Schleweinsky (2006) for a more elaborated distinction) and a process of structural reanalysis correlated with the activation of the centro-parietal area, the so called P600.

It is commonly accepted that electrophysiological signatures are not topologically well-defined. According to Zurif, data from Broca's patients (that is, subjects with a lesion in the left anterior areas) could help to define the spatial dimension. In his proposal, a finer functional topography of the brain has to reconcile neuropsychological data with processing evidence. It is possible that much evidence from aphasia and some

principles elaborated as parsing strategies could be unified in a more powerful explanatory model. This proposal is in line with our assumption and in the next section we will present an explanation in a similar vein.

"For the present however, - as Zurif points out - *the similarity of these accounts must be emphasized, not their few differences. It should be apparent that Hickok, and Grodzinsky before them, all agree on what is particularly problematic for Broca's patients; namely, the inability of these patients to represent intra-sentence relations involving traces and their resultant inability to understand non-canonical sentences in which constituents have been extracted from object position"*.

2. Grammatical principles as parsing strategies

In the present chapter we present experimental data on M.R.'s comprehension of relative clauses and aim to show the advantages of integrating processing-based accounts with representational approaches to agrammatism. Moreover, with data from sentence processing we provide support for our views concerning the grammatical nature of natural language processing.

We claim that the subject in the present case study makes use of certain (grammatical) distinctions, which are marginal in normal processing, to help build up the correct syntactic representation and arrive at the relevant interpretation of complex sentences. We claim that this evidence provides support for the idea that certain grammatical principles, in this particular case those governing locality, are indeed general principles of optimal computation applying at different levels of mental representation and giving rise to similar patterns in intact and impaired systems.

It is not sufficient to address agrammatism as a selective problem with non-canonical sentences; instead, a more suitable instrument seems to be the adoption of more general principles of syntactic structures. The advantage of this approach is that it can directly explain the way in which different elements are integrated in the syntactic structure.

The first formulation of this deficit in terms of syntactic chain formation was proposed by Grodzinsky (1990) in his influential Trace Deletion Hypothesis (TDH henceforth). His proposal has been the object of much discussion, but it has the indisputable merit of having introduced formal linguistic description into the study of agrammatic aphasia.

Grodzinsky's idea is that comprehension deficits in agrammatic aphasia can be reduced to a deficit in the construction of syntactic dependencies between moved elements and their traces, since traces are not represented in Broca's patients (see Grodzinsky 1990, 2000 for details). His main argument relates to the syntactotopic conjecture, where essential syntactic principles have a correlate in brain structures.

One important implication of this proposal is a systematic correlation between linguistic entities (such as traces, a special kind of empty category) and brain regions. This argument has been disproved in many studies (see the extensive commentary in Grodzinsky, 2000), which have shown that Broca's aphasics do produce sentences with traces in them and that many overlapping brain regions are involved in their processing. This apparent incongruence is predicted by a purely representational model, such as Grodzinsky's. Certain aspects of the TDH need to be looked at in greater depth in order to better understand the approach presented in this study. Grodzinsky claims that not all syntactic competence is lost in agrammatic aphasia, but only a very specific part of it. Agrammatic patients should be incapable of representing traces as these are deleted and their interpretations are not recoverable in the syntactic representation. Without traces there will be no way of connecting the moved elements to their original positions and assigning them their original thematic roles. If an experiment involves an irreversible sentence subjects should be capable of recovering the thematic information required by the task (*Who did what to whom?*) from other systems external to the core grammar. In the case of reversible sentences, agrammatic patients would apply a non-grammatical cognitive strategy by which they assign the agentive theta role to the first NP encountered. This strategy gives positive results when the first NP of the sentence does indeed bear the agentive theta role (subject relatives, subject clefts, etc.), but generates a chance level (or non-standard) performance when the first NP does not bear the agentive theta role (object relatives, object clefts, passives, etc.).

The co-occurrence of trace deletion, which impedes the transmission of the correct theta role to the displaced NP, and the extra-grammatical strategy [NP1= Agent] seems to correctly predict the agrammatic comprehension pattern.

But this approach to language impairment does not tell us how linguistic information is integrated in the structure, and consequently why the trace could have a different neurocognitive implementation. According to Grodzinsky's description of agrammatic comprehension, an interaction is established between an incomplete grammatical representation and a non-grammatical heuristic [NP1= Agent]. The first-agent strategy applies only in the case of an NP that has not received a thematic role by grammatical analysis. So, a purely syntactic condition, [-ϑ], governs selection of the elements to which the strategy applies. In processing terms, this means that the application domain of the strategy can only be defined once a syntactic analysis has been made. That is to say, only after failure of thematic role assignment is it possible to use the strategy. This heuristic is necessary in a comprehension task, where the subject must assign thematic roles.

Furthermore, Grodzinsky does not provide any direct connection between the TDH and a possible Working Memory deficit (many studies have ascribed deficits in working memory to impairments in Broca's area; see, for example, Just and Carpenter, 1992); although it is possible that such a connection exists, in line with some important work by Zurif, Swinney and others (see Zurif et al. 1993).

Many revisions of the TDH have been proposed in the literature. For example, Hickok and Zurif (1993) claim that agrammatic patients are capable of understanding structures in which at least one theta role is assigned locally (without the mediation of a trace) because they maintain the knowledge of the theta-grid associated with each verb.

Hickok and Zurif (ibidem) present evidences relevant to the Trace Deletion Hypothesis. They tested comprehension of subject relatives in sentences such as (94).

(94) *The child who combs the mother is blond*

The subject was asked to answer the question *"Who is blond* ? ".

The TDH predicts a non-impaired performance on subject relatives, yet aphasic participants in this study performed at chance level. This sort of evidence showing a deficit in the comprehension of subject relatives is not predicted by the extra-grammatical strategy put forward in the TDH. Difficulties in comprehension emerge when two possible NPs compete for an unassigned thematic role. Chance level performance was found with structures such as that exemplified in (95)[2].

(95)[The child]$_i$ [$_{CP}$ who[$_{VP}$ [**t**]$_i$ combs the mother]] [$_{VP}$ [**t**]$_i$ is blonde]

To formulate their approach on agrammatic comprehension they introduce the notion of *thematic assignment representation* (T.A.R.). This is exemplified for the verb 'to comb' in 96.

(96) " Comb (x (y))"

---

[2] It would be interesting to test the same empirical paradigm manipulating other features. In Italian it is possible to test a gender mismatch between arguments with sentences such as: *Il bambino che pettina la mamma è biondo* 'The child (m) who combs the mother (f) is blonde (m)'.

where x denotes the thematic role assigned to the external argument, i.e. the subject, and y the role assigned to the complement. An impaired T.A.R. of the subject relative is presented in (97); the asterisk represents an unassigned thematic role caused by incorrect computation.

(97) Combs (* (the mother))
is blonde (*)

The verb to comb does not assign the external argument a thematic role as this is mediated by a trace (in this formulation they follow the VP-internal subject hypothesis). Only the local role of the complement of the transitive verb is not trace-mediated, and so grammatically assigned.

The thematic role of the predicate "is blonde" has two possible candidates (both the NPs are still in the input system). Comprehension is not impaired if there is only one possible candidate for an unassigned thematic role. Under experimental conditions where the subject is forced to assign thematic roles performance is at chance level with configurations such as (95).

This is interesting, in large part because it is not necessary to involve an extra-grammatical strategy based on the canonical order of thematic roles.

Furthermore, it correctly supports the notion of thematic role assignment as a strongly local phenomenon. Hickok's proposal is that the agrammatic comprehension pattern involves the ability to establish an antecedent–trace relation in the syntactic analysis of the sentence.

For an exhaustive presentation of the Revised TDH (RTDH) see Hickok, Zurif and Canseco-Gonzalez (1993), which also contains an interesting discussion on the validity of Grodzinsky's experimental methodology.

In our proposal we have an initial indication of a complexity effect induced by the presence of two possible governors of a dependency, but in Hickok, Zurif & Canseco-Gonzalez's (ibidem) proposal the impairment has a representational source, in line with Grodzinsky's assumptions on trace. No connection with a possible processing source of the deficit is clearly formulated.

In a recent study on comprehension in aphasia (Grillo, 2003, 2005 and 2008), there is an explicit attempt to unify the two approaches sketched above and reduce the comprehension asymmetries (in particular those between comprehension of sentences with canonical vs. non-canonical word order) to a special case of Minimality Effects.

Grillo proposes that the loss of (syntactic) processing abilities can compromise the representation of the full array of morphosyntactic features normally associated with syntactic elements, thus giving rise to Minimality Effects in precise syntactic configurations (see also Garraffa and Grillo, 2008). As presented in the previous chapter regarding production, an impoverishment of the syntactic representation can reduce the environment in which syntactic relations are allowed, making it impossible for the agrammatic patient to construct certain 'long distance' relations. I will summarize those aspects of this approach necessary for understanding the present study.

According to Relativized Minimality (RM) (Rizzi, 1990), in an abstract configuration like (98) a local structural relation cannot hold between X and Y if Z is a potential bearer of the relevant relation and Z intervenes between X and Y.

(98) X…Z…Y

So, for instance, the local relation linking a moved phrase to its trace holds in (99c), but not in (99b)[3]: The *Wh* operator *who* intervenes between *how* and its trace in (99d), and since *who* is a potential bearer of the antecedent relation the required antecedent-trace relation fails, and the question is ungrammatical.

(99) a How did you solve the problem?
b How did you solve the problem **t**?

(99) c I wonder who could solve the problem in this way
d * How do you wonder *who* could solve this problem **t**?

Rizzi (2001) shows that the possibility of forming a chain between X and Y depends on the nature of the elements involved and more specifically on the set of morphosyntactic features associated with each element.

(100) … X … Z … Y
[α,β,γ,δ,ε] [α,β,γ,δ] [α,β,γ,δ,ε]

In (100) a particular set of morphosyntactic features is associated with every node.

[3] Examples from Rizzi (2001).

We may think of this set of features as the specification of grammatical information: i.e. phi features (number, gender), case, thematic roles, grammatical category.

A crucial point, but not within the scope of the present investigation, is related to the possible order of this information. This is the object of much discussion in theoretical linguistic models.

Given this configuration, RM allows the formation of a relation, a syntactic chain, between X and Y: the presence of the element **ε** suffices for RM to *see* the difference between X and Z and therefore to authorize the movement of Y over Z (**ε** should be thought of as the distinctive feature of the particular head and the relevant relation we are considering, i.e. a [*wh-*] feature in the head of a FocP, which if missing would imply a change of "class" of the relevant set from Argumental to Quantificational). The reader is referred to Grillo's article and to Rizzi (2004) for the original formulation of Minimality effects in terms of classes of features.

Grillo (ibidem) claims that a possible cause of aphasics' limited processing capacity is that they are not always able to maintain activation of the representation of all the morphosyntactic features normally associated with syntactic nodes. Thus some of the features needed for the computation of structures involving dependencies over possible interveners may be absent.

(101) ... X ... Z ... Y
$[\alpha,\beta,\gamma,\delta]$ $[\alpha,\beta,\gamma,\delta]$ $[\alpha,\beta,\gamma,\delta]$

This leads us to expect an asymmetry in aphasics' treatment of dependencies: those involving one NP "crossing" over another should be more problematic than those that don't. The asymmetry between aphasic comprehensions of object movement (which implies crossing of the subject NP) vs. subject movement (which doesn't imply crossing of any NP) supports this hypothesis.

The main difference between the constructions tested is related, in fact, to the presence or absence of a potential intervener between the moved element and its trace. Subject questions are correctly predicted not to be problematic; no NP intervenes between the moved subject and its trace. No Minimality Effects are expected even if the syntactic representation is impoverished.

This approach to aphasic comprehension and in general to grammatical deficit has many interesting consequences for the formulation of an organic theory on the grammatical nature of linguistic processing. For example, in many works on sentence processing there is an explicit reference to the concept of complexity (see Just and Carpenter, 1998).

To define what is complex in sentence processing we need to refer to syntactic theory. Otherwise, the best we could hope to achieve would be a list of structures ordered by their complexity judged according to empirical measures. We will thus know which structures are easier and which are more difficult to process, but we will not know why this is so, nor will we have a definition of complexity, merely a description.

On the basis of RM, in fact, we can provide a definition of complexity in terms of the number and quality of morphosyntactic features which need to be maintained as active in the syntactic representation in order for the computation not to crash. On the same basis we will put forward a hypothesis on the nature of the comprehension deficit in agrammatism that can predict which structures are more difficult for patients to understand.

Furthermore, reducing comprehension and production patterns in aphasia to general principles limiting the availability of different syntactic representations in unimpaired adult systems allows us new questions concerning the nature of those principles and of the system itself.

If we want to build a complete theory of aphasia we also need to know why certain constructions are more complex than others. We believe that the only way to reach this goal is to define the potential effects of limitations in processing capacity at the representational level and to get rid of any generic definition of complexity. To this end, we will present some interesting data on processing and possible parsing strategies in line with the present approach.

Many experiments on sentence processing have reported slower reading times in sentences with an NP NP V order, such as 102b, compared with NP V NP order, 102a (Schrifers, Friederici and Kuen,1995; Gibson,1998; De Vincenzi, 1991).

(102a) NP V NP The teacher who greets the student …
(102b) NP NP V The teacher who the student greets …

Interesting evidence comes from a corpus of Dutch and German texts (Vonk and Sheiefers, 2002). The main finding of this study is that there is no difference in reading times between subject and object relatives when the object is inanimate. Animacy seems to influence the processing of relative clauses. A mismatch in terms of animacy appears to be an important cue for the parser. This data is partially comparable with the evidence on WH production in the previous chapter.

It is important to bear in mind that this effect is related to the syntax of the clause and not to a possible disturbance in thematic role assignment.

A recent study on object agreement in Basque (Erdozia, Laka et al., 2009) reports a clear electrophysiological effect, specifically a left anterior negativity (LAN) at the verb position in OSV order but not in SOV order. This was tested by presenting an experimental paradigm with ambiguous chains.

(103) Emakume**ak** gizon**ak** ikusi ditu
Woman-the Sub/Obj man Sub/Obj seen has
The woman has seen the men **or**
The man has seen the woman

In (103) one of the constituents is the singular subject of the sentence while the other is the plural object. As OSV is a possible order, without any prosodic information the sentence is ambiguous. At the verb position, these sentences elicit a frontal negativity related to syntactic reanalysis. Furthermore, in non-ambiguous OSV sentences displaced constituents elicit a LAN while the verb elicits a P600.

(104) Emakumeak gizonek ikusi dituzte
Woman –the Sbj/Obj man Sbj seen have
The men have sees the women

The sentence in (104) starts ambiguously (the first constituent could be the subject or the object) but the second constituent, whose morphology shows it to be the subject of the sentence, disambiguates it.

This research provides additional support for the idea that displaced elements increase syntactic complexity and hence increase the processing cost of a given sentence. In other words, there is an additional cost for long dependencies.

This approach to language parsing is compatible with a parsing principle, the Minimal Chain Condition, elaborated by De Vincenzi (1991). The basic formulation, based on her extensive study of Italian, is summarized below.

(105)
Minimal Chain Condition (MCC):
Avoid postulating unnecessary chain members, but do not delay required chain members.
(De Vincenzi,1991)

The second part of the principle may be couched in terms of another parsing principle elaborated by Frazier (1999).

(106)
Active Filler Hypothesis:
Once an element of the category XP is identified as moved from its argument position, then posit a corresponding empty XP category as soon as the grammar of the language allows you to do so.

In this case, posit the shortest chain at any given argument position.

Some interesting data emerges in De Vincenzi's study on Italian dependencies. In chapter 2 we presented data concerning the difference between unaccusative and unergative subjects. Another interesting phenomenon came to light in the investigation of temporary ambiguity in the comprehension of interrogatives. Slower reading times were recorded for (107b) than for (107a). In Italian the preferred interpretation of (107a) is with a subject in first position. This indicates that the system prefers to resolve an ambiguity by establishing the shortest chain.

(107a)Chi ha contattato il poliziotto?
Who has called the policeman?

(107b)Chi hanno contattato i poliziotti?
Who have called the policemen?

Thus there is a preference for a 'subject first' analysis, but then the morphology reveals that the item in first position, *chi*, is in fact an object.

We want to conclude this section with a comment on the nature of chains as real linguistic objects.

An element such as the interrogative operator in the sentences in (108) below '*must receive both the interpretive property "patient of the verb read" and the interpretive properties "interrogative", "topic", "focus", respectively:*

(108) a. Which book did you read _?
b. This book, you should read_?
c. THIS BOOK you should read_! (rather than those crappy comics) (from Grillo 2005)

Natural languages express this duality of interpretive properties by having the phrase occur in two positions, each assigning one kind of property. In standard terminology, an element is moved from a position of one kind to a position of the other kind' (Rizzi 2004c).

As is pointed out in Grillo's work, the ban on movement results from Minimality; the breakdown of a chain impedes the understanding of '*this duality of interpretive properties'*. An open chain is not a syntactic object, i.e. it cannot express this duality; thus Topics, relative pronouns and interrogatives are emptied of any thematic property and so the aphasic subject doesn't know who did what to whom.

In the present work we will explain the data collected from M.R.'s comprehension of relative clauses invoking grammatical principles that affect the normal processing of non-canonical sentences, for example, the preference for minimal chains resulting from an incompletely specified feature set. The aim of this approach to grammatical deficit is to bring agrammatic aphasia into the realm of purely grammatical description and to highlight the grammatical basis of sentence processing.

3. The study

In this paragraph we review the results of different sentence comprehension tasks (language screening + the present experiment) to provide a background to analysis of M.R.'s performance on the comprehension of relative clauses. As shown in the introductory paragraph on M.R.'s language screening, in the case of standard reversible relative clauses M.R. performs well above chance level (85%) on *subject relatives* and at chance level (40%) on *object relatives*. This result is in line with the picture emerging from cross-linguistic evidence (see Grodzinsky, 2000 and related works).

A second experiment was run to investigate the influence of mismatches in agreement features between subject and object.

In English, subject and object relative clauses (RCs) are disambiguated by word order: subject RCs display the canonical SVO order, while object RCs display a non-canonical OSV order.

In Italian, the sentence "Il ragazzo che ha salutato il maestro" (lit. The boy that has greeted the teacher) is an ambiguous sentence. Il maestro could be either the object of the relative clause or the post-verbal subject.

Agreement feature on the verb can disambiguate this type of sentence as in "I ragazzi che hanno salutato il maestro" (lit. The boys that have greeted the teacher) where *il maestro* is the post-verbal subject of the relative clause, or as in *I ragazzi che ha salutato il maestro* (The boys that has greeted the teacher) where *il maestro* is the object of the relative clause. Object relatives can also have the following word order *I ragazzi che il maestro ha salutato* (lit. The boys that the teacher has greeted).

We tested whether comprehension of object relatives would be less problematic when the arguments of transitive verbs, the subject and the object, were distinguished in number features.

Furthermore, we investigated mismatches in agreement and position as possible aids to interpreting non-canonical structures in a system typically impaired with respect to the comprehension of object relative clauses. By testing object relatives with a VS order, as in *I ragazzi che ha salutato il maestro*, we investigate the predicted preference for a minimal chain over the morphological cue.

The subject took part in a picture selection task testing non-ambiguous object relatives. The experimental items were:

a. 40 object relatives with pre-verbal subject;
b. 40 object relatives with post-verbal subject.

We administered the test twice, thus obtaining 80 items for each type. Number agreement of both arguments was balanced. Non-semantically reversible sentences (e.g. Il ragazzo che dipinge il quadro è biondo, The boy who paints the picture is blond) were used as fillers. The results are summarized in the table below.

	RC	**Mismatch**	**Inversion**	**Correct**	**Sentences**
A	**Subject**	-	-	34/40 85%	The boy that has greeted the teacher
B	**Subject**	+	-	72/80 90%	The boy that has greeted the teachers
C	**Object**	+	+	38/80 47.5%	The boy that have greeted the teachers
D	**Object**	+	-	59/80 73.7%	The boy that the teachers have greeted
E	**Object**	-	-	16/40 40%	The boy that the teacher has greeted
(A)	**Object**	-	+		
	Total			219/320 68.4%	

Table 21. M.R.'s performance on the comprehension of relative clauses in a picture selection task

A mismatch in agreement features on the verb clearly helps the patient in the construction of the relevant chains. This is evident if we compare object relatives such as in D and E in table 21.

M.R. performed at chance level in the comprehension of object relatives with post-verbal subjects (type C) 42/80, 52.5% (p0.525 $\chi(1)=0.2$). Object relatives with pre-verbal subjects differ significantly from those with post-verbal subjects ($\chi(1)=11.5464$ $p<0.05$).

Comprehension of object relatives with pre-verbal subjects shows a high error rate: 21/80, 26% (p 0.2625, $\chi(1)=18.05$ $p<0.05$). Subject relatives are above chance (85% and 90%), even though there is a significant deviation from standard performance.

In object relatives with mismatched agreement and crossing of an argumental position, as in D, we still have a significant number of errors, 21/80 (26%).

Object relatives with pre-verbal subjects are less impaired than those with post-verbal subjects.

Ambiguous object relatives give rise to a chance performance, with only 40% correct responses; unambiguous object relatives are correctly understood more than 70% of the time.

An important question at this point is: *how is it that certain distinctions between antecedents and intervening elements, such as agreement mismatch, that do not seem to count in the normal grammar seem to play such an important role in positively influencing the performance of an impaired subject?*

As a preliminary answer to this question suffice it to say that regardless of the impairment the system seems to work in exactly the same way: if enough distinctions are visible the chain can be built; if not then the derivation crashes. In the normal case certain distinctions are not relevant for minimality: the presence of higher order features that have already marked the relevant elements as belonging to a particular class (somehow categorizing it) is all that the system has to look at. But if such distinctions are not available the system can adapt and resort to other distinctions to get the work done.

We thus consider that the evidence from relative clause comprehension supports the analysis proposed here.

4. Discussion: on the grammatical nature of processing

The differences between relatives with pre-verbal subjects and those with post-verbal subjects highlight the importance of making more fine-grained distinctions in the impaired system: differences in number features do not play a role in normal language processing (probably due to the presence of higher order features); they do, however, play a role in an impaired system in helping to cross a potential intervener (D vs. E in Table 21).

A mismatch in agreement features on the verb clearly helps the patient in the construction of the relevant chain. Ambiguous object relatives give rise to chance performance, with only 40% correct responses (see D); unambiguous object relatives are correctly understood more than 70% of the time (see E). This provides yet further evidence to support the view that agreement is a strong feature in establishing a chain (compare also B vs. C); otherwise object relatives, as in C, would be assigned a wrong subject interpretation, so that they would be parsed as subject relatives, as in B.

The presence of a pre-verbal subject in the relative clause [NP-NP-V-gap] forces M.R. to revise her decision and the sentence is interpreted using agreement morphology.

Revision of a post-verbal clause, such as C [NP- (gap)-V-NP-gap], takes place at the embedded verb. At this point a memory-impaired system will probably delete material.

Relative clauses with the subject in post-verbal position, as in C, show the *Minimal chain condition* (De Vincenzi, 1991) is being applied.

In the case of temporary ambiguity the system prefers to posit a shorter chain. After the relative pronoun the system closes the dependencies in the gap position

(109) The boy that have greeted the teachers…
X … Z (Agr) … Y

Only after the verb is there revision in favor of a subject interpretation, as indicated by the morphological marker.

The crucial difference between this assumption and an account such as Trace Deletion is that we are assuming the presence of a syntactic chain between the elements X and Z. This is not directly tested in the present study, since we did not make an on-line analysis of the sentence. It could be the object of a future study in which possible priming effects in position Z, indicating the presence of the chain, would be tested.

The present approach on acquired language disorders makes precise predictions regarding the nature of the reduced procedural capacities of aphasics and is compatible with parsing models that posit *on-line* construction of a syntactic representation in language production (De Vincenzi; 1991; Friderici, 1992 and Swinney et al, 1993). The parser's preferences will be tied to both the structural characteristics of the sentence and to the predictions of the parsing principle. Another important aspect to the interpretation of our results in terms of a reduction of processing capacity is De Vincenzi's (1991) *Minimal Chain Condition* .

We should expect limitations in forming chains over an intervening element where there is a reduction in the number (and quality) of features associated with each syntactic node.

In processing obligatory filler-gap constructions (such as relative clauses) the parser prefers to close the dependency and form a grammatical object: a syntactic chain. The differences between relative clauses with pre-verbal subjects and those with post-verbal subjects show the importance of making more fine-grained distinctions in the impaired system: differences in number features, which do not play a role in normal language (probably due to the presence of higher order features), do play a role in impaired grammars in helping to cross a potential intervener.

However, comprehension of object relatives with mismatched agreement shows 26% errors. This result can be explained in terms of *Locality Effects*.

The approach presented in Grillo (2005; paragraph 2) identifies an impoverishment in the number and quality of morphosyntactic features associated with syntactic nodes as a source of the problem with non-canonical clauses.

(110)... X ... Z ... Y ...
$\{\alpha,\beta,\gamma,\delta\}_{\text{class A}}$ $\{\alpha,\beta,\gamma,\delta\}_{\text{class A}}$ $\{\alpha,\beta,\gamma,\delta\}_{\text{class A}}$

This underspecification is the consequence of a limitation in (syntactic) processing capacities. Chance level performance in object relatives and a high percentage of errors in unambiguous object relatives are possible consequence of a reduced grammatical specification but compatible with general principles on syntactic representations such as locality

However, an underspecified system is nonetheless subject to general principles of the grammatical system such as locality effects, and parsing strategies such as the Minimal Chain Condition.

An approach in terms of reduced information regarding a given grammatical principle, such as the locality condition, is more appropriate under the view that procedural capacity has a grammatical nature.

Furthermore, well-known problems such as cross-patient variability or the varying complexity of different syntactic strings are not difficult to overcome, since underspecification can be structurally defined.

This line of thinking has certain consequences for real-time processing. It is usual to suppose that in a syntactic dependency relation the antecedent constituent is held in a memory buffer until it receives a thematic interpretation in its argument position. Thus a lexical item must be activated twice, in two different positions.

This basic intuition needs further refining.

Interesting evidence in support of syntactic processing as an expression of formal linguistics comes from an ERP experiment on German (Felser et al., 2003). This study reports different components in topicalized sentences from those in interrogatives. Both structures elicit a Left Anterior Negativity (LAN), a general indication of the presence of a dependency and measure of an extra load in working memory. This component is more prominent in *Wh* dependencies. These results support the idea that different syntactic dependencies are processed differently, distinguishing Topics from *Wh* operators.

These issues may be better addressed via language-related brain potentials techniques applied on patients with cortical and sub-cortical left hemisphere lesions (see, for example, Friederici, von Cramon and. Kotz, 1999) in a productive interdisciplinary environment where data on lesions are the compendium for a timing model expressed with brain potentials. In Friederici et al.'s study, patients with lesions in the left frontal cortical and sub-cortical areas and in the basal ganglia (a possible deeper area source of the grammatical deficit) were tested on auditorily presented sentences with semantic and syntactic violations and asked to make grammaticality judgments. Event-related potentials and reaction times were recorded and compared with normal controls. Three different components correlated with different language processes were considered: the N400, assumed to reflect processes of semantic integration; the ELAN, associated with initial syntactic structure building; and a late positivity P600. In normal participants the expected N400 component for semantically incorrect sentences was elicited, while an early anterior negativity followed by a P600 was elicited for syntactically incorrect sentences. In patients with left frontal cortical lesions, however, an attenuated N400 component was elicited in the semantic condition. In the syntactic condition, only a late positivity was observed. Patients with lesions of the basal ganglia, in contrast, showed an N400 for semantic violations and an early anterior negativity along with a P600 for syntactic violations, similar to normal controls. Under the assumption that the early anterior negativity reflects automatic first-pass parsing processes and the P600 component more controlled second-pass parsing processes, the present results suggest that the left frontal cortex, but not the basal ganglia, may be involved in early parsing processes in sentence comprehension.

This study is crucial for the present approach since it presents evidence for a more clearly defined localization of cortical functions related to early syntactic processing.

Zurif et al. (1993) carried out priming experiments on the comprehension of sentences with syntactic dependencies, such as (111).

(111)The gymnast loved the professor from the north-western city who complained about the bad coffee.

Normal subjects show faster reaction times to a word semantically related to the antecedent ('the professor from the north-western city') presented after *who* (for example, "the teacher") than to an unrelated word, indicating that the antecedent is reactivated in this position. A similar facilitation, however, was not found with aphasic subjects, indicating that they do not reactivate the antecedent.

The data analyzed here, and more importantly the general difficulty with so called non-canonical structures shown in cross-linguistic studies on aphasia, seem to provide consistent support for a strict correlation between grammar and parsing strategies.

The problems with non-canonical structures encountered by agrammatics arise from the fact that in these structures an element similar to the moved antecedent intervenes between the latter and its trace, impeding formation of the syntactic object that is the very essence of movement by blocking chain construction. It is important to stress that this mechanism applies in exactly the same way as it applies in 'normal' grammars. In fact, in a non-trivial sense there is no difference between aphasic and normal grammars; at the relevant level of analysis it makes no sense to speak of agrammaticism at all.

CHAPTER SEVEN

A DERIVATIONAL APPROACH TO LOCALITY CONDITIONS IN THE LIGHT OF APHASIA

The case study presented here concludes that M.R.'s linguistic deficit is a grammatical restriction due to impoverishment of procedural capacities. Her impairment may be interpreted in terms of a reduction compatible with general principles of phrase structure.

Our argumentation is couched mainly in terms of theoretical linguistics but we think it is also necessary to bear in mind the cognitive implementation of phrase structure building. In the present study we have not investigated M.R.'s language processing, although the conclusions reached regarding her linguistic abilities have implications for real-time processing.

The hypothesis put forward by Zurif (1980) is that Broca's patients suffer from a central deficit involving all language modalities. The nature of the impairment is syntactic and the linguistic performance of their patients is defined as "asyntactic". It follows from this that the processing of syntactic information is instantiated in those cortical areas found to be damaged in Broca's aphasics (Zurif, 2001).

Unfortunately, studies of linguistic deficits do not provide a clear picture from which to infer the neural organization of language. Influential proposals include localization models (such as Grodzinsky's Trace Deletion Hypothesis), variable localization models (such as many studies reported by Caplan where different areas of the brain support the same functions in different subjects), even distribution models (such as Damasio and Damasio's (1992) whose hypothesis is that large regions of the brain equally support a range of functions) and uneven distribution models (Mesulam, 1990).

None of these models formulates a clear set of methodological constraints within which to study the language of aphasic patients. In our opinion this is in part related to the selection of the grammatical phenomenon that is the object of investigation and in part related to the brain imaging technique, not at the moment a suitable instrument to investigate language. Interesting evidence comes from the interaction of brain potentials techniques integrated with localization information coming from the patient's data (as presented in chapter 4).

In the present study we have presented various data supporting the view that aphasics have a deficit in the formation of syntactic dependencies (see also Garraffa and Grillo,2008). De Vincenzi also found slower processing of syntactic dependencies in her extensive work on Italian (De Vincenzi, 1991). Furthermore, we show that aphasic subjects, as in the present case study, offer the possibility to investigate reduction in the activation of grammatical information, and their performance could be crucial for studying the different quality of dependencies related to different features present in sentences.

In this approach we mainly seek to describe a limitated processing capacity as a source of the deficit. Many studies have ascribed impairments in Broca's area to deficits in working memory (see, for example, Just and Carpenter, 1992); it is possible that such a connection exists, in line with some important work by Zurif, Swinney and others (see Zurif et al. 1993).

Friederici and Frazier (1992) proposed that agrammatic comprehension is not a deficit of general verbal memory capacity but of processing demands imposed by "structural inference chains". In their study, they elaborated the Complexity Limitation Hypothesis.

(112) Complexity Limitation Hypothesis:
Principle 1: The grammar is intact.
Principle 2: Input rate, memory span and computational speed are related. A complete constituent structure may be accurately assigned to a sentence only if sufficient resources are available to syntactically structure the input string roughly as the individual items appear.
Principle 3: The thematic processor is intact.

They stated that the impairment in agrammatic Broca's aphasics could be attributed to *"the loss of automaticity of syntactic parsing [...] by automaticity we mean the fast, well-coordinated characteristic of over learned skills. The loss of automaticity in syntactic parsing and the resulting conscious syntactic processes seem to cause a high sensitivity to syntactic violations".*

To integrate the two approaches, representational and processing accounts, we need to better describe the nature of linguistic processing in relation to constraints already specified in natural languages. To address this issue we will interpret some well-established evidence from Broca's aphasia in term of processing strategies as the Minimal Chain Condition (De Vincenzi, 1990) elaborated in the domain of sentence processing.

1. Syntactic parsing principles: on the limits of computations

In the literature on sentence parsing strategies we can trace a long history of investigations underlining the role of grammatical analysis in sentence processing. Parsing principles and principles of grammar often show strong similarities, and grammatical principles have often been proposed (also) on the basis of processing considerations (as in binary branching, or antisymmetry). However, the most common situation is one in which, despite the similarity, a distinction is still needed to distinguish between the two, the former generally capturing 'preferences', while the latter involved in grammaticality. One of the first models proposed to describe syntactic parsing was the garden path model (Frazier and Fodor, 1978), in which universal processing strategies compatible with every natural language are assumed to play a role in sentence parsing. The study of these strategies has allowed for the elaboration of certain principles, which are able to describe the preferences of the syntactic parser in an incremental fashion. Some of these principles are well-known, such as Minimal Attachment (MA) and Late Closure (LC)[1].

In the last forty years many data have been collected in various languages and the application of these principles has been widely discussed, essentially because these preferences seem not to hold cross-linguistically and/or depend on extra-syntactic conditions (such as pragmatic factors and plausibility on a non-linguistic level).

It is not a trivial matter to integrate the specificities of natural languages into a model of syntactic parsing without losing the universal character of its descriptive principles, since these cross-linguistic differences may be grammaticalized in the languages concerned.

Processing strategies (such as MA and LC) are conceived as being not so much language-specific as motivated by cognitive factors, such as memory limitations. The logical alternative is that extra-grammatical factors (for example, frequency or plausibility) may be considered

---

[1] Minimal Attachment: *Attach incoming material into the phrase marker being constructed using the fewest nodes consistent with the well-formedness rules of the language under analysis.*
Late Closure: *attach an incoming component to the phrase currently being processed, if grammatically permissible.*

edifying strategies for the parser, but the model as such will not in any sense be informative about the computations necessary to build a sentence.

Many other principles and parsing models have been proposed over the years to describe various linguistic phenomena. For example, many psycholinguistic studies have investigated filler-gap relations. An effect detected during the syntactic processing of these linguistic relations was formalized by Frazier as the Active Filler (Frazier, 1987).

(113) Active filler: *once an element of the category XP is identified as moved from its argument position, then posit a corresponding empty XP category as soon as the grammar of the language allows you to do so.*

It is not within the scope of the present article to give an exhaustive picture of parsing principles and models in relation to syntactic analyses. The present introduction serves to present the Minimal Chain Principle, on which we intend to base our discussion.

2. Processing non-local dependencies: a sketch of MCC

Marica De Vincenzi aimed to further the study of parsing strategies with data from a Null-Subject language, Italian, and investigation of specific properties of this language.

Regarding the processing of empty categories in Italian, De Vincenzi proposed a novel principle, the Minimal Chain Condition (MCC), which unifies the processing of different kinds of empty categories (De Vincenzi, 1991).

(114) Minimal Chain Condition:
a. *avoid postulating unnecessary chain members;*
b. *but do not delay required chain members.*

The MCC was proposed as a consequence of De Vincenzi's investigation of empty categories in Italian and in particular of the occurrence of null subjects, the differences between various licensing conditions, and certain properties of interrogative pronouns.

As far as the present article is concerned, we wish to point out that the main advantage of the MCC principle is that the specification of conditions on chain formation (locality conditions) has a direct link with linguistic principles. Previous syntactic parsing principles have had no direct relationship with theoretical evidence. The idea embodied in the

MCC is that processing mirrors the form of the linguistic representation.

We wish to propose a specification of the MCC through investigation of the grammatical system of aphasics and the different strategies adopted by this population to establish syntactic dependencies. The topic is crucial in specifying the nature of a non-fully-fledged parser (presumably affected by processing limitations), neither in terms of extra-grammatical strategies, nor in terms of a 'good enough' heuristic approach. On the contrary, by re-specifying the MCC principle, we wish to provide support for a generalized mechanism that is more efficient in aphasia due to the ability to detect minimality effects.

As previously mentioned, the Minimal Chain Condition was formulated as a result of an extensive investigation of empty categories in Italian (De Vincenzi, 1991). In particular, the study investigated the cost involved in building syntactic chains in different configurations, such as post-verbal subjects and the filler–gap relation in interrogatives. Differences in processing empty categories in Italian can be explained by the MCC, as it characterizes the behavior of the parser in terms of distance.

Testing adults' reading times on declarative sentences with post-verbal subjects, De Vincenzi has shown that VS structures with unaccusative verbs (such as (115a)) were easier to process than structures containing unergatives (such as (115b)).

(115a) E' arrivato un bambino
Is arrived a child
A child has arrived
(115b) Ha esitato un bambino
Has hesitated a child
A child hesitated

With the lexically expressed indefinite NP subject in post-verbal position the structures with unaccusative and unergative verbs differ in the length of their chains. Several linguistic analyses assume direct thematic role assignment to the subject of an unaccusative verb. According to this view, the subject of an accusative verb is a surface direct object (see Belletti, 2001). Only unergative verbs need to establish a dependency in order to link the two positions for assignment of the thematic role. With unaccusatives, chain formation is not required and the grammatical subject in object position does not share any pronominal feature with the pre-verbal subject position. This evidence strongly supports the hypothesis that chain formation is a costly process for the human sentence parser.

Interesting data regarding Italian dependencies were reported in De

Vincenzi's investigation of temporary ambiguity in the comprehension of interrogatives. Slower reading times were recorded for sentences such as (116b) than for (116a). In Italian the preferred interpretation of (116a) is that of subject in first position, indicating that the system prefers to resolve an ambiguity by establishing the shortest chain.

(116a) Chi ha contattato il poliziotto?
Who has called the policeman?
(116b) Chi hanno contattato i poliziotti?
Who have called the policemen?

There is, therefore, a preference for a 'subject first' analysis. However, in (116b) the verb morphology reveals that the item in first position, *chi*, is in fact an object. At this stage, processing a revision (due to the interference of object agreement) is costly for the parser.

Many experiments on sentence processing have reported slower reading times in sentences with non-canonical word order, such as Object-Subject-V order in an object relative clause (117b) compared with Subject-V-Object order in a subject relative clause (117a) (Schrifers, Friederici and Kuen, 1995; Gibson, 1998; De Vincenzi, 1991; among others).

(117a) Subject V Object: The teacher who greets the student is gentle
(117b) Object Subject V: The teacher who the student greets is gentle

This pattern, often called the canonicity pattern, shows that sentences with canonical argument orders, as in (117a), are easier to process than sentences with non-canonical order.

Non-canonical reversible sentences require further syntactic computation. These findings have also been recorded in very distinct grammars and the processing mechanism may, therefore, be universal. This canonicity pattern has been recognized in many natural languages and implies the availability of a universal parsing strategy rather than different properties related to word order in specific languages.

As De Vincenzi's data show, this is not only a consequence of the canonical ordering of arguments (a principle such as the active filler would be enough to explain this effect). The distance between the elements involved in the dependency to be computed also plays a role.

Following the spirit of the MCC in processing obligatory filler-gap constructions (such as relative clauses) the parser prefers to close the dependency and form a grammatical object: a syntactic chain. This approach explains the way in which various elements are integrated into the syntactic structure.

The data presented can be interpreted in terms of the MCC but it should be pointed out that there is a precise grammatical motivation for invoking this principle. While the second part of the principle may be couched in terms of the active filler parsing principle elaborated by Frazier, the conditions involved in the first part can be explained in terms of a calculation based on features, as we will see in the next section.

It is clear that there are further costs in processing sentences with non-canonical order and there could, therefore, be a preference for discarding these patterns. This kind of reasoning may seem paradoxical, since in natural languages displacement of phrases is pervasive.

Assuming that a syntactic structure is characterized by a particular computation of ordered elements, it is of no interest to compile a list of complex sentences or a gradient of complexity in itself. It is preferable to start from what is present in natural languages and the specific needs of syntactic computation, and for this reason we are interested in studying aphasia as a window onto properties that are difficult to identify in normal sentence processing.

3. MCC and Minimality

Performing a linguistic task involves assignment of thematic roles, but where factors of complexity intervene Broca's aphasia patients can make the wrong assignment, as we saw in chapter 6. The mechanism can be directly explained by De Vincenzi's MCC principle.

In Grillo's approach to aphasia an explicit attempt was made to reduce comprehension asymmetries (in particular, comprehension of sentences with canonical vs. non-canonical word order) to a special case of Minimality Effects.

The loss of (syntactic) processing abilities can compromise the representation of the full array of morphosyntactic features normally associated with syntactic elements, thus giving rise to Minimality Effects in precise syntactic configurations (see also Garraffa and Grillo, 2008).
This leads us to expect an asymmetry in aphasic treatment of dependencies: those involving one NP crossing over another similar one should be more problematic than those that don't. The asymmetry between aphasic comprehension of object movement (which implies crossing of the subject NP) vs. subject movement (which doesn't imply crossing of any NP) supports this hypothesis.

The main difference between the constructions tested is, in fact, related to the presence or absence of a potential intervener between the moved element and its trace. Subject questions are correctly predicted not to be problematic: no NP intervenes between the moved subject and its trace. No Minimality Effects are expected even if the syntactic representation is impoverished. This approach to aphasic comprehension and to grammatical deficit in general has many interesting consequences for the formulation of a formal theory of the grammatical nature of linguistic processing. For example, in many works on sentence processing there is explicit reference to the concept of complexity (see Just and Carpenter, 1998). To define more clearly what complexity in sentence processing is, we need to refer to syntactic theory. Otherwise, the best we could hope to achieve would be a list of structures ordered by their complexity judged according to empirical measures. We will thus know which structures are easier and which are more difficult to process, but we will not know why this is so, nor will we have a definition of complexity, merely a description.

On the basis of RM, in fact, we can provide a definition of complexity in terms of the number and quality of morphosyntactic features which need to be maintained as active in the syntactic representation in order for the computation not to crash. On this basis, we will propose a hypothesis on the nature of the comprehension deficit in agrammatism that can predict which structures are more difficult for patients to understand. This is expressed by Grillo in (118).

> (118) Generalized Minimality,GM : *Given any instance of non-local movement (i.e. movement that inverts the base order of constituents) underspecification of the feature structure of a moved element X can generate a minimality effect whenever X crosses an element Y whose featural specification is consistent with that of X.*

Underspecification can be caused by any (permanent or temporal) reduction of syntactic processing capacities. We claim that GM captures the same set of phenomena as the MCP and bridges the gap between parsing preference and grammaticality in a natural way, which completes the MCP.

The rationale behind GM is that the full representation of the morphosyntactic feature structure of a syntactic constituent has a processing cost and that a computational system driven by (among other factors) economy considerations might try to avoid those costs. This perspective has the major advantage of reducing well-known asymmetries in complexity between subject and object movement (and in availability in the case of agrammatic aphasics, young children, or adult speakers in stressful situations) to a special case of Relativized Minimality.

(119) Generalized Minimality / MCC:
a. Avoid postulating unnecessary feature structure
b. Do not delay the representation of required feature structure

(119) clearly corresponds to (114a): postulating additional unnecessary feature structure means postulating additional chain members; i.e. if we take the DP the girl in "*Show me the girl . . .*" to be the head of a relative clause (therefore representing the DP with a [+rel] feature) the parser is by definition postulating an unnecessary chain member (i.e. a two member chain, leaving aside unnecessary details on intermediate positions) between the position in CP which heads of relative clauses move to and the original extraction position. There is therefore a clear correspondence between representing features of a certain kind, e.g. quantificational, discourse-related features, and representing additional chain members. The same similarity applies to the second conjunct of the two principles (119b and 114b). Delaying the representation of required feature structure implies delaying the representation of required chain members: a delay in the representation of a [+rel] feature on the head of a relative clause implies that the chain member in CP will not immediately be represented, with predictable consequences once the parser encounters evidence for the necessity of the postulation of those features/chain members. An advantage of the formulation in terms of feature structure is that not only do we expect a preference for the closest gap, on the basis of minimality, but we can predict in what kind of environments the preference will turn into a mistake expressed in terms of a minimality effect.

This approach has the clear advantage of treating mistakes as structures ruled out by grammatical principles. Generation of featurally impoverished syntactic structures allows us to rule them out on a par with other more standard cases of syntactic violation[2].

The character of the serial human sentence processor the MCP supports is directly expressible in terms of minimality, a pervasive property of the sentence. The rationale for the MCP is psychological, and it could be related to restriction in short-term memory capacity during a time pressure task. A solution to performing this task is to group information in structured units. Miller (1956) demonstrated that the more structured the material to be remembered the less burden it places on

[2] This conception of mistake is in line with much work on error as the result of the application of standard 'correct' operations to underspecified data structures (see Reason, 1990, for an overview of the relevant literature).

memory. For language it means that unstructured verbal material is more costly to store in memory.

To build a complete theory of aphasia we need to know why certain constructions are more complex than others. We believe that the only way to reach this goal is to define the potential effects of the limitations in processing capacities at the representational level and to get rid of any generic definition of complexity.

An approach in terms of reduced information on a given grammatical principle, compatible with parsing strategies, is more appropriate from the view that procedural capacity has a grammatical nature. Furthermore, well-known problems such as cross-patient variability or the varying complexity of different syntactic strings are not difficult to overcome, since the processing costs could be structurally defined.

An interesting way to address this point could be a systematic study of so-called mismatch effects in grammatical and ungrammatical sentences, to investigate the nature of different grammatical cues. As we see in this study mismatch in agreement features between argument in relative clauses and mismatch in animacy in WH dependencies are a crucial cue for establishing the correct representation-interpretation in a damaged system. This intuition could be brought back to a grammatical principle for distinguishing the features' implementation.

For example, a possible grammatical distinction could be made between Head-marking languages (or argument-marking), languages where cases of animacy are overtly expressed and Agreement-marking languages. In this sense there could be a sort of variation to distinguish the different strategies.

A natural field of investigation to place side by side with the pathological data is the study of development of grammatical strategies. Interesting data in the acquisition domain reveals a possible maturational effect of principles such as the Minimal chain condition, compared with agreement mismatches, which first appear as soon as syntactic structures are testable in children (see Arosio, Adani and Guasti, 2010).

Cross-linguistic comparison could show interesting preferences, as in French, where subject relatives are less costly to process even in the presence of an agreement marking on the complementizer (see Frauendfelder et al., 1980).

This kind of evidences opens up the possibility of investigating models of grammatical features where different information is integrated in a preferential order, as the one hypothesized in (120).

(120) $S > O_{animacy}\ O_{pos} > O_{morph}$

To conclude, the core idea of this study is that language processing has an intrinsically grammatical basis. Syntactic principles, such as locality conditions, refer directly to on-line sentence processing. In this sense, processing is a grammatical analysis in a serial system implemented in the brain. A convergence of data from neurolinguistics, sentence-processing and the acquisition domain support this view of the language faculty.

BIBLIOGRAPHY

Anton Mendez, I., 1996 *Clitics and attraction errors* M.A. thesis University of Arizona.

Arosio, F., Adani, F., and Guasti, M.T. 2005 *Processing grammatical features by Italian children,* (eds.) David Bamman, Tatiana Magnitskaia and Collen Zaller. Proceedings of the 30th Boston University conference on Language Development.

Avrutin, S. 1999 *Development of the Syntax-Discourse Interface*. Kluwer Academic Publishers, Dordrecht, The Netherlands.

—. 2000a *Comprehension of discourse D – linked and non D - discourse linked WH questions by children and Broca's aphasics*. In Grodzinsky, Y., Shapiro, L. P. and Swinney, D.A. (eds.), *Language and the brain: Representation and Processing.* (pp.295-312). San Diego: Academic Press.

—. 2000b *Language acquisition and language impairments: a comparative psycholinguistic approach.* Brain & Language, 71, 7-9.

—. 2001 *Linguistic and agrammatism.* GLOT International Vol.5 n.3.

—. 2004 *Weak syntax*. Ms. Utrecht University.

Baker, M.C. 1988 *Incorporation: A theory of grammatical function changing*. Chicago, IL: University of Chicago Press.

Bastiansee, R., et al., 2002 *Verbs: some properties and their consequences for agrammatic Broca's aphasia*. Journal of Neurolinguistics 15, 239-264.

Benedt, M. J., et al., 1998 *A cross-linguistic study of grammatical morphology in Spanish and English speaking agrammatic patients.* Cortex, 34:309-336.

Belletti, A., 2000 *Agreement Projections,* in M. Baltin and C. Collins(eds.) *The Handbook of Syntactic Theory,* Blackwell.

—. 2001. *"Inversion as Focalization*". In A. Hulk & J. Y. Pollock, (eds). *Inversion in Romance and the theory of Universal Grammar* pp.60-90). Oxford University Press.

—. 2002 *Structures and Beyond. The Cartography of Syntactic Structures.* Vol.3., Oxford University Press.

Belletti, A., Bennati, E., and Sorace, A., 2007 *Theoretical and developmental issues in the syntax of subjects: evidence from near-native Italian"*, Natural Language and linguistic Theroy 25: 4 657-689.

Becker, M., 2000 *The acquisition of the copula in child English. The lightness of be.* PhD dissertation UCLA.

Benedet, M. J., Christiansen, J. A., Goodglass, H. 1998 *A cross-linguistic study of grammatical morphology in Spanish- and English-speaking agrammatic patients. Cortex,* 34, 309-336.

Berntzen, K., and Hestivick, A., *2003 Movement vs. Tree size as predictor of difficulty for agrammatics: evidence from Norwegian dialects.* Proocedings for Science of aphasia conference, SOA04 Trieste.

Bock, K. and Miller C.A., 1991 *Broken agreement.* Cognitive Psychology 23, 45-93.

Bock, K. and Eberhard, K. M. 1993 *The meaning, sound, and syntax of English number agreement.* Language and Cognitive Processes, 8, 57-99.

Bock, K., and Cutting, J. C., 1992 *Regulating mental energy: Performance units in language production.* Journal of Memory and Language, 31, 99-127.

Bornkessel, I., and Schlesewsky, M. 2006 *Introduction to event-related brain potentials in language research.* Materials for the AIPS Seminar school. Bertinoro 2007.

—. 2006 *The Extended Argument Dependency Model: A Neurocognitive Approach to Sentence Comprehension across Languages.* Psychological Review, 113 (4), 787-821.

Brandi, L. and Cordin, P. 1989 *Two Italian dialects and the null subject parameters.* In O. Jaeggli and K. Sapir (eds.) *The null subject parameter.* Kluwer Academic Publishers Dordrecht, pp.111-142.

Brown, M., Keurs, T. and Hagoort, P. 1999 *Electrophysiological signatures of Visual Lexical Processing: Open-and Closed-class words.* Journal of Cognitive Neurosciences, 11:3 pp 261-281.

Caplan, D., 1987 *In defense of agrammatism.* Cognition, 24: 273-76.

—. 1995 *The cognitive neuroscience of Syntactic Processing,* in Gazzaniga, M. S. *The cognitive neurosciences.* Cambridge MA: MIT Press. 871-879.

—. 2001 *The Measurement of Chance Performance in Aphasia, with Specific Reference to the Comprehension of Semantically Reversible Passive Sentences: A Note on Issues Raised by Caramazza, Capitani, Rey, and Berndt (2001) and Drai, Grodzinsky, and Zurif (2001).* Brain & Language 76.2, 193-201.

Caplan, D. and Futter, F. 1986 *Assignment of thematic roles to nouns in sentence comprehension by an agrammatic aphasic.* Brain & Language 27:117-134.

Caplan D. and Hildebrandt, N. 1988 *The man left without traces: a case study of aphasic processing of empty categories.* Cognitive Neuropsycology 4 : 257-302.

Caplan, D. and Waters, G. S., 1996 *Verbal working memory and sentence comprehension.* Brain & Behavioural Science, 22: 77-126.

Caramazza, A., 1990 *Cognitive neuropsychology and neurolinguistics: advances in models of cognitive function and impairment.* New Jersey: Lawrence Publishers.

—. 1997 *How many level of processing are there in lexical processing?* Cognitive Neuropsychology 14: 177-208.

Caramazza, A., and Zurif, E. B., 1976 *Dissociation of algorithmic and heuristic processes in language comprehension. Evidence from aphasia.* Brain & Language 3: 572-82.

Caramazza, A., Capitani, E., Rey, A. and Berndt, R. S., 2001 *Agrammatic Broca's Aphasia Is Not Associated with a Single Pattern of Comprehension Performance.* Brain & Language 76.2, 158-184.

Caramazza, A., and Shapiro, K., 2004 *Language Category in the brain. Evidence from aphasia.* In Belletti A., *Structures and beyond: The cartography of Syntactic structures*, Vol.3 OUP.

Cardinaletti, A. and Starke, M. 1999 *The typology of structural deficiency: a case study of the three classes of pronouns.* In *Clitics in the language of Europe*,ed. Henk van Riemsdijk, 145-233. Berlin: Mouton de Gruvter.

Chierchia, G., and Guasti, M. T., 2000 *Backwards vs. Forward Anaphora: Reconstruction in Child Language,* Language Acquisition, 8.2:129-170.

Chinellato, P. 2002 *Agreement disorder, subject clitic and the structure of IP in dialectal agrammatism: The Field Damage Hypothesis.* Cortex 38: 837-40.

—. 2002 *Analisi linguistica e nuove strategie riabilitative in neurolinguistica: alcuni casi di agrammatismo dialettale.* Manoscritto Università di Padova.

Chomsky, N., 1981 *Lectures on Government and Binding.* Dordrecht: Foris Publications.

—. 1995 *The Minamilist Program.* Cambridge MA: MIT Press.

—. 2000 *Su natura e Linguaggio*. a cura di Luigi Rizzi e Adriana Belletti . (eds.) Edizioni Università di Siena.

—. 2005 *Three factors in language design.* Linguist Inquiry: vol.36, n 1.

Cinque, G. 1990 *Types of A'-Dependencies*. Cambridge MA: MIT Press.
—. 1999 *Adverbs and functional heads*. New York: Oxford University Press.
—. 2002 *Functional Structure in DP and IP. The Cartography of Syntactic Structures, vol.1*. New York: Oxford University Press.
Cresti, D. 1995 *Extraction and Reconstruction* Natural Language Semantics, 3, 79-122.
De Vincenzi, M., 1991 *Syntactic parsing strategies in Italian*. Holland: Dordrecht, Kluwer.
De Vincenzi, et al., 2003 *Differences in the perception and time course of syntactic and semantic violations*. Brain and Language, 85 (2): 280-296.
De Vincenzi, M., et al., 2010 *Mapping the language: A reading time and a topographic ERP study on tense, agreement, and Aux–V violations.*. In Rosalia Di Matteo and Luca Tommasi (eds.) *Cross-linguistic perspectives on language processing* . John Benjamins Publishing company.
Doron, E., 1988 *On the Complementarity of Subject and Subject-Verb Agreement*. In Michael Barlow and Charles A. Ferguson (eds.) *Agreement in Natural Language: Approaches, Theories, Descriptions*. Stanford: CSLI.
De Bleser, R., Luzzatti, C., 1994 *Morphological processing in Italian agrammatic speakers: syntactic implementation of inflectional morphology*. Brain & Language 46:21- 40.
Drai, D., Grodzinsky, Y., and Zurif, E., 2001 *Broca's Aphasia Is Associated with a Single Pattern of Comprehension Performance: A Reply* . Brain & Language 76.2, 185-192.
Drai D., Grodzinsky, Y. 2006 *A new empirical angle on the variability debate: Quantitative neurosyntactic analyses of a large data set from Broca's Aphasia*. Brain & Language 96.2, 117-128.
Drai D., Grodzinsky, Y. 2006 *The variability debate: More statistics, more linguistics*. Brain & Language, 96.2, 157-170.
Erdozia, K., and Laka, I., 2009 *Syntactic complexity and ambiguity resolution in a free word order language: behavioral and electrophysiological evidences from Basque*. Brain & Language 109.1, 1-17.
Felser C., Clahsen, H., and Münte, T. 2003 *Storage and integration in the processing of filler-gap dependencies: an ERP study of topicalizations and wh-movement in German*. Brain and Language, 87, 345-354

Fernandez, E. M. 2007 *Effects of ambiguity resolution caused by the timing of RSVP presentation emulate effects caused by explicit prosody*. Abstract for CUNY07.

Ferreira, F. and Clifton, C. 1986 *The independence of syntactic processing*. Journal of memory and language, 25, 348-368.

Ferreiro S. 2003 *Root infinitives in child and agrammatic Ibero-romance: presence vs. absence of the phenomenon*. Manuscript Universitat Autònoma de Barcelona

Frank, J., Lassi, G., Frauenfelder, U. H. and Rizzi, L., 2006. *Agreement and movement: syntactic analysis of attraction* Cognition, 101, 173-216.

Frauenfelder, U. H., Segui, J., and Mehler, J. 1980 *Monitoring around the relative clause*. Journal of Verbal Learning and Verbal Behavior, 19, 2.

Frazier, L. 1987 *Processing Syntactic Structures: Evidence from Dutch*. Natural Language Processing and Linguistic Theory, 5, 519-559.

Frazier, L., and Friederici, A., 1991 *On deriving the properties of agrammatic comprehension*. Brain and Language, 40, 51-66.

Frazier, L., and Friederici, A., 1992 *Thematic analysis in agrammatic comprehension: syntactic structures and task demands*. Brain and Language, 42, 1- 29.

Friederici, A., 2002 *Towards a neural basis of auditory sentence processing*. Trends in cognitive Sciences, 6:22, 78 - 84 .

Friederici, A., Hickok, G. & Swinney, D. 2001 *Brain Imaging and Sentence Processing* (a Special Issues) Journal of Psycholinguistic Research, 30 (3).

Friederici, A., and Kilborn, K. 1989 *Temporal constraints on language processing: Syntactic priming in Broca's aphasia*. Journal of Cognitive Neuroscience, 1, 262 – 272 .

Friederici, A., 1995 *The time course of human syntactic activation during language processing*. Brain and Language, 50, 259 – 281.

Friedmann, N., 1994 *Morphology in Agrammatism: a dissociation between Tense and Agreement*. Thesis M.A. degree in Cognitive Psychology Tel Aviv University.

—. 1998 *Functional categories in agrammatism: a cross linguistic study*. PhD dissertation Tel Aviv University

—. 2000 *Moving verbs in agrammatic production*. In Bastiaansee, R., and Grodzinsky, Y., (eds.) *Grammatical disorders in aphasia: a neurolinguistic perspective*. London: Whurr.

—. 2001 *Agrammatism and The pscicologycal reality of the syntactic tree*. Journal of Psycholinguistic Research, Vol.30, No.1.

—. 2002 *Question production in Agrammatism: The tree Pruning Hypothesis.* Brain & Language 80:160-187

Friedmann, N. and Grodzinsky, Y. 1997 *Tense and Agreement in Agrammatic Production: Pruning the syntactic tree*. Brain & Language 56:397- 425.

—. 2000 *Split inflection in neurolinguistics*, in M. A. Friedmann, L. Rizzi (eds.) *The acquisition of Syntax: issues in comparative developmental linguistics.* London: Longman Linguistics Library.

Friedmann, N., Shapiro, L. P. 2003 *Agrammatic comprehension of simple actives sentences with moved constituents: OSV and OVS structures.* Journal of Speech language and hearing research 46,288-297.

Garraffa M. 2003 *Linguistica e deficit grammaticale: studio di un caso.* Unpublished thesis, Università di Siena.

—. 2004 *Task dependence effects: What are you asking for? A good context for eliciting WH questions.* Poster presented at Science of Aphasia V conference. Potsdam, Berlin.

Garraffa, M. and Grillo N. 2008 *Generalised minimality. Canonicity effects as a grammatical phenomenon.* Journal of Neuroliguistic 21, 177- 197.

Garraffa, M. and Lorusso, P. 2008 *Verb Classes and Subject Distribution in Italian.* Abstract presented at the Internationl conference Romance turn 2, Utrecht University.

Garraffa, M., 2009 *Minimal structures in aphasia: a study on agreement and movement in a non-fluent aphasic speaker.* Lingua: 119:10, 1444 - 1457.

Garraffa, M., Di Domenico, A. and Di Matteo, R. 2010 *The syntactic domain of number agreement: attraction effects and pronominal classes.* In Servidio E. and Moscati V. (eds.) CISCLWP, vol. 4 MIT Press Cambridge MA.

Garrett, I., 1980. *Levels of processing in sentence production.*In B.Butterworth (eds.), Language Production: 1 San Diego Academic Press.

Gavarrò, A., and Martinez, S., 2002 *Tense and Agreement impairment in Iberian languages*. Journal of Psycholinguistics research, vol. 36:1, 25 – 46.

Guasti, M. T., and Rizzi, L., *Agreement and Tense as distinct syntactic positions.* In Guglielmo, Cinque (eds.) *The structure of DP and IP.* Oxford University Press.

Gibson, E., 1998 *Linguistic complexity: Locality of syntactic dependencies.* Cognition, 68, 1-76.

Grillo, N., 2003 *Agrammatic comprehension between processing and representation – minimality effects*. Unpublished Thesis, Università di Siena.

—. 2005 *Minimality effects in agrammatic comprehension*. Proceedings of XIV Console. Blaho, S., Schoorlemmer, E., Dicente, L. (eds.)

—. 2008 *Generalised minimality*. PhD dissertation Utrecht Institute of Linguistics,OTS.

Grodzinsky, Y. 1990 *Theoretical perspective on language disorder*. Cambridge, MA: MIT Press.

—. 1995 *A restrictive theory of agrammatic comprehension*. Brain & Language 50,27-51.

—. 2000 a *The neurology of Syntax: language use without Broca's area*. Behavioural and Brain Science 23 (1): 47-117.

—. 2005 *Syntactic dependecies as memorized Sequences in the Brain*. Canadian Journal of Linguistics, special 50th anniversary issue.

Grodzinsky, Y., and Reinhart, T., 1993 *The innateness of binding and coreference*. Linguistic Inquiry 24, pp. 69-101.

Grodzinsky, Y., Shapiro, L. P., and Swinney, D.A., 2000 *Language and the Brain: Representation and Processing*. Academic Press, NY.

Hamman, C. and Belletti, A., 2008 *Developmental patterns in the acquisition of complement clitic pronouns: comparing different acquisition modes with an emphasis on French*. Rivista di Grammatica Generativa , 31, 39-78.

Hartsuiker, R. J., and Kolk, H. H. J., 2001 *Error monitoring in speech production: A computational test of the perceptual loop theory*. Cognitive Psychology, 42 (2), 113-157.

Hagiwara, H. 1995 *The breakdown of functional categories and the economy of derivation*. Brain & Language, 50 : 92-116.

Haarmann, H. J., Just, M. A. and Carpenter, P.A. 1997 *Aphasic sentence comprehension as a resource deficit: a computational approach*. Brain & Language 59:76-120.

Haarmann, H. J. and Kolk, H. H. J. 1992 *The production of grammatical morphology in Broca's and Wernicke's aphasics. speed and accuracy factors*. Cortex 28:97-102.

Heycock, C., and Krok, A., 1999 *Pseudocleft Connectivity: Implications for the LF Interface*. Linguistic Inquiry 30.3: 365-397.

Heycock, C., and Zamparelli, R., 2005 *Friends and colleagues: Coordination, plurality, and the structure of DP*. Natural Language Semantics 13: 201-270.

Hickok, G., Zurif, E. and Canseco-Gonzales, E. 1993 *Structural description of Agrammatic Comprehension*. Brain & Language 45:371-395.

Heim, I., 1987 *Where does the definiteness restriction apply?* In Eric Reuland (eds.) *The Representation of (In) Definites*. Cambridge, Mass.: MIT Press.

Hickok, G., and Avrutin, S., 1995 *Comprehension of WH questions by two agrammatic Broca's aphasics.* Brain & Language, 51: 10-26.

Hillert, D. and Swinney, D. 2001 *The processing of fixed expressions during sentence comprehension.* In Cienki, A., Luka, B.J., & Smith, M.B. (Eds.), *Conceptual and Discourse Factors in Linguistic Structure*, CSLI Publications, Stanford, Ca., 107-122.

Jakobson, R. 1957 *Shifters, verbal categories, and the Russian verb.* Cambridge, Mass.: Dept. of Slavic Languages and Literatures, Harvard University.

Just, M. A. and Carpenter, P.A. 1992 *A capacity theory of comprehension: individual differences in working memory.* Psychological Review 99:122-149.

Kayne, R., 1991 *Romance clitics, verb movement and PRO.* Linguistic Inquiry 22.4: 647-86.

Kolk, H. H. J. 1998 *Disorders of syntax in aphasia, linguistic –descriptive and processing approach.* In B. Stemmer and H. Whitaker (eds.) *Handbook of Neurolinguisitc.* Academic Press, San Diego.

Kuperberg,G., Caplan D, Sitnikova T, Eddy M, Holcomb PJ. 2006 *Neural correlates of processing syntactic, semantic and thematic relationships in sentences.* Language and Cognitive Processes 21(5): 489-530.

Lorusso,P. 2003 *L'.acquisizione dei verbi inaccusativi.Studio sulla produzione spontanea dei parlanti.* MA dissertation Università di Siena.

Lorusso, P., Caprin, C. and Guasti, M.T. 2005 *Overt subject distribution in early Italian children.* Supplement proceedings of BUCLD04 conference.

Luzzatti, C., A. Toraldo, and Guasti, M.T. 2001 *Comprehension of reversible active and passive sentences in agrammatism. Aphasiology 15(5)*: 419-41.

Marinis, T., 2000 *The acquisition of clitic objects in Modern Greek: Single Clitics,Clitic Doubling, Clitic Left dislocation.* ZAS Paper in Linguistics, 15, 2-23.

Mak, W. M., Vonk, W., and Schriefers, H. J. 2002. *The influence of animacy on relative clause processing.* Journal of Memory and Language, 47 (1), 50-68.

Mauner, G., Fromkin, V. and Cornell, T. 1993 *Comprehension and acceptability judgment in agrammatism: disruption in the syntax of referential dependency.* Brain and Language 45, 340-370.

Menn, L. and Obler, L., 1990 *Agrammatic Aphasia. A Cross-Language Narrative Sourcebook*, Amsterdam/Philadelphia: J. Benjamins Publishing.

Miceli, G., Burani, C., Capasso, R. and Laudanna, A. 1994 *Batteria per l'analisi dei deficit afasici - B.A.D.A.* CEPSAG, [2nd ediction].

Nespoulous, J.L. et al., 1988 *Agrammatism in sentence production without comprehension deficits: reduced availability of syntactic structures and/or grammatical morphemes?* Brain & Language 33:273-295.

Neuhaus, E., and Penke,M., 2003 *Question production in German Broca's aphasia.* Brain and Language, 87:59-60.

Neville, H.J., Mills D.L. and Lawson D.S. 1992. *Fractionating language: different neural subsystems with different sensitive periods.* Cerebral Cortex, 2(3), 244-58.

Nicol,J. and Swinney, D. 2001 *Special Issue on Human Sentence Processing: CUNY 2000* Journal of Psycholinguistic Research Part I : 29 (6) and Part II: 30 (1).

Osterhout, L. 2000 *On space, time and language for the next century, timing is (almost) everything.* Brain and Language 71,175-177.

Osterhout,L., Kim, A. and Kuperberg, G., 2009 *The neurobiology of sentence comprehension.* In M. Spivey, M. Joanaisse, & K. McRae (Eds), *The Cambridge Handbook of Psycholinguistics.* Cambridge: Cambridge University Press.

Pearlmutter, et al., 1999 *Linear versus hierarchical agreement feature processing in comprehension.* 12th CUNY conference, NY.

Pollock, J. Y. 1989 *Verb movement , universal grammar and the structure of IP.* Linguistic Inquiry 20: 365 -424.

Reznik, M., and S. Dubrovsky. 1995 *Agrammatism in Spanish: a case study.* Brain and Language *51* 355-68.

Rizzi, L. 1990 *Relativized Minimality.* Cambridge, MA: MIT Press.

—. 1997 *The fine structure of the left periphery.* In *Elements of grammar.* edited by Haegmann L., Dordrecht: Kluwer.

—. 2000 *Reconstruction, Weak island sensitivity and Agreement.* Ms. Università di Siena.

—. 2002 *Relativized Minimality effects.* In Baltin and Collins C., The handbook of Syntacitic theory . Blackwell,Oxford.

—. 2004a *Locality and the left Perifery.* Belletti A. (eds.) Structures and Beyond. The cartography of Syntactic Structures, Vol.2, Oxford University Press.

—. 2004 b *The structure of CP and IP. The cartography of syntactic structures* . Vol.3 Oxofrd University Press.

—. 2004c *On the form of chains: criterial positions and ECP effects.* Ms Università di Siena.

Roberts, I. 1987 *The representation of implicit and dethematized subjects.* Foris -Dorderecht.

Roberts, I. 1993. *Verbs and diachronic syntax.* Dordrecht: Kluwer

Ross, J. R. 1969 *Guess Who?* In Binnick R., Davison A., Green G. and Morgan J. (eds.) Papers form the 5th regional meeting of the Chicago linguistic society 252-286. Chicago Linguistic society: Chicago III.

Ruigendijk, E., Kouwenberg, M., and Friedmann, N. 2004 *Question production in Dutch agrammatism.* Brain and Language, 91, 116-117.

Ruigendijk, E., S. Baauw, S. Zuckerman, N., Vasic, J., de Lange and Avrutin, S., (to appear). *A cross-linguistic study on the interpretation of pronouns by children and agrammatic speakers: Evidence from Dutch, Spanish and Italian.* To appear in: E. Gibson & N. Pearlmutter (Eds.) Processing and Acquisition of Reference.

Schriefers, H., Friederici, A. and Kühn, K, 1995 *The processing of local ambiguous relative clauses in German.* Journal of Memory and Language, 34, 499-520.

Stavrakaki, S., and Kouvava, S., 2003 *Functional categories in Agrammatism: Evidence from Greek.* Brain and Language 86(1), 129-141.

Stowe, L. A. 1986 *Evidence for on-line gap location.* Language and Cognitive Processes 1:227-245.

Swinney, D., and Fodor, J. D. 1989 *Introduction for the Special issue.* Journal of Psycholinguistic Research.18, (1), 5-19.

Szabolcsi, A., 1999 *Strong and weak islands. Syntax companion,* Case study n.102, University of Utrecht.

Thornton, R., 1995 *Referentiality and Wh-movement in Child English: Juvenile Delinkuency.* Language acquisition: 4, 139-175.

van der Meulen, I., 2004 *Syntactic movement and comprehension deficits in Broca's aphasia* LOT Dissertation Series 95.

Vespignani, F. 2006 *Agreement violations.* Manuscript Università di Padova.

Watanabe, A., 2006 *In WH movement: moving on.* Edit Lisa Cheng and Norbert Cover. MIT Press.

Waters, G. S., and Caplan, D., 1996 *The capacity theory of sen-. tence comprehension critique of Just and Carpenter.* Psychological Review, 103, 1–12.

Wenzlaff, M. and Clahsen, H. 2004 *Tense and Agreement in German agrammatism.* Brain and Language 89:57-68.

Zurif, E.B., Swinney, D., Pratter P., Solomon J., Busher C. 1993 *An on-line analysis of syntactic processing in Broca's and Wernicke's aphasia.* Brain and Language 45, 448-464.

Zurif, E.B., and coll. 1995 *Brain regions of relevance to syntactic processing.* In L.Gleitman and M.Liberman (eds.), *An Invitation to Cognitive Science*, Vol. I. Cambridge, MA:MIT Press [2nd ediction].

Zurif, E.B., 1980. *Language mechanics: a neuropsychological perspective.* American scientist: 68, 305–311.

Zurif, E.B., 2001 *More on sentence comprehension in Broca's aphasia: A response to Caplan.* Brain and Language, 79, 321-328.

—. 2000 Review of "*Handbook of Neurolinguistics*" (B. Stemmer and H.A. Whitaker, eds.). Applied Psycholinguistics, 21, 557-566.